Caring for People with
Learning Disabilities

Caring for People with Learning Disabilities

Edited by:

IAN PEATE

Associate Head of School, School of Nursing and Midwifery, University of Hertfordshire

DEBRA FEARNS

Senior Lecturer, School of Nursing and Midwifery, University of Hertfordshire

John Wiley & Sons, Ltd

Other Wiley Editorial Offices

John Wiley & Sons Inc., 111 River Street, Hoboken, NJ 07030, USA
Jossey-Bass, 989 Market Street, San Francisco, CA 94103-1741, USA
Wiley-VCH Verlag GmbH, Boschstr. 12, D-69469 Weinheim, Germany
John Wiley & Sons Australia Ltd, 42 McDougall Street, Milton, Queensland 4064, Australia
John Wiley & Sons (Asia) Pte Ltd, 2 Clementi Loop #02-01, Jin Xing Distripark,
Singapore 129809
John Wiley & Sons Canada Ltd, 6045 Freemont Blvd, Mississauga, ONT, L5R 4J3

Wiley also publishes its books in a variety of electronic formats. Some content that appears
in print may not be available in electronic books.

Library of Congress Cataloging-in-Publication Data

Caring for people with learning disabilities / edited by Ian Peate, Debra Fearns.
  p. cm.
  Includes bibliographical references and index.
  ISBN-13: 978-0-470-01993-1 (pbk. : alk. paper)
  ISBN-10: 0-470-01993-X (pbk. : alk. paper)
1. Learning disabilities. 2. Learning disabled – Services for. I. Peate, Ian. II. Fearns,
Debra.
  LC4818.L435 2006
  371.9 – dc22
                                                                      2006011246

A catalogue record for this book is available from the British Library

ISBN-13: 978-0-470-01993-1
ISBN-10: 0-470-01993-X

Typeset by SNP Best-set Typesetter Ltd., Hong Kong
Printed and bound in Great Britain by TJ International Ltd, Padstow, Cornwall

This book is printed on acid-free paper responsibly manufactured from sustainable forestry
in which at least two trees are planted for each one used for paper production.

Dedication

I would like to dedicate this book to the many adults with learning disabilities I have had the pleasure to meet and work with over the years, who have enriched my life and taught me patience, understanding and compassion. The students I have taught have given me hope for the future of learning disability nursing and continue to inspire me.

Debra Fearns

I dedicate this text to all those who strive to ensure fairness in the delivery of healthcare for all members of society.

Ian Peate

Contents

About the Editors

Ian Peate, EN(G) RN DipN (Lond) RNT BEd(Hons) MA(Lond) LLM
Ian began his nursing a career in 1981 at Central Middlesex Hospital, becoming an Enrolled Nurse working in an intensive care unit. He later undertook three years' student nurse training at Central Middlesex and Northwick Park Hospitals, becoming a Staff Nurse then a Charge Nurse. He has worked in nurse education since 1989. His key areas of interest are nursing practice and theory, sexual health and HIV/AIDS. He is currently Associate Head of School. His portfolio centres on recruitment and marketing and professional academic development within the School of Nursing and Midwifery.

Debra Fearns, BA (Hons), RNLD, MA, Post-graduate Diploma in Teaching and Learning
Debra Fearns is a Senior Lecturer in the School of Nursing and Midwifery at the University of Hertfordshire. She is a Registered Nurse (Learning Disabilities), and teaches on Learning Disability nursing across pre- and post-registration courses. Debra completed an MA in Health and Social Policy in 1998. The dissertation focus was centred on how Custody Officers recognise vulnerability, especially in people with learning disabilities. The research was carried out in a Shire police force. Publications include *Appropriate Adults and Appropriate Adult Schemes: Service User, Provider and Police Perspectives,* Ed: Brian Littlechild (2001), published by BASW, Venture Press and Debra has recently jointly edited *Mental Disorder and Criminal Justice: Policy, Provision and Practice* (2005) with Brian Littlechild, published by Russell House Publishing Ltd.

Contributors

Frank Garvey, RNMH, RGN, RNT, BA (Hons), Cert Ed, Cert Health Ed
Frank has worked in the fields of learning disability and general nursing for 25 years. Within that time he has been a charge nurse; a respite care home manager for children with complex medical needs and learning disabilities; a community learning disabilities nurse and a university senior lecturer involved in the education of nurses and social workers. He is particularly interested in the physical healthcare of people with learning disabilities and in the research of attitudes towards disability.

Currently, Frank works for Hertfordshire Partnership Trust (HPT) at a strategic level, promoting the equitable healthcare of people with learning disabilities when they are being cared for within general hospitals. He also leads on research development for the learning disability nurses within HPT and on the development of the Expert Patient Programme (EPP) in Hertfordshire for people with learning disabilities.

April Hammond, BSc (Hons), Nurse Specialist Practitioner, Community Learning Disabilities, RNMH, Senior Lecturer Hertfordshire University
April originally worked in a respite care setting for children and adults with learning disabilities. She then became a Community Nurse and Health Facilitator for people with learning disabilities and worked in four London boroughs, before taking up her current post as a Senior Lecturer for student learning disability nurses and student social workers. April's specialist interests are women's health, sexual health and relationship issues. She is particularly passionate about the welfare and rights of people with learning disabilities and keenly encourages service users' involvement in training student nurses.

Costas Joannides, BA, DipHE
Costas is a Placement Support Nurse (Learning Disabilities) working for Hertfordshire Partnership NHS Trust. He has supported and worked within Learning Disability practice for 20 years. His clinical interests are challenging behaviour, reflective practice, education and quality assurance. Costas comes from a family of nurses and educators so nursing has always been part of his life.

Outside of work his interests are restoring lambrettas to their former glory, collecting vinyl (northern soul) and managing a Sunday football team.

Jackie Kelly, MA, PgDip, Registered Nurse in Learning Disability, Academic/ Professional Group Leader, Senior Lecturer Learning Disability

Since commencing her career in learning disability nursing in 1987, Jackie has worked in a variety of contexts. Her work has provided diverse opportunities to work with and learn from people with a wide range of needs and experiences, as well as with their families. Jackie remains constantly grateful and humbled by the privilege of sharing such experiences. As a community nurse she became interested in the *whole family* experience of having a person with a learning disability within the family. This interest led to her undertaking a Masters in Applied Systemic Theory, giving her the opportunity and the tools to explore these connections from a systemic perspective. This has been invaluable both in her work with people with learning disabilities and in her teaching. Teaching within the University has been an exciting opportunity to convey this systemic viewpoint within the context of nurse and social work education. As part of Jackie's studies she carried out a small piece of empirical research exploring the experiences of siblings of a person with a learning disability. This remains a research interest, which she hopes to further develop in the future.

Paul Maloret, RNLD, Dip HE, BA(hons), PGCE

Paul's interest in working with people with learning disabilities was generated from an unforeseen situation. At the age of 18, like so many people of a similar age in the early 1990s, Paul headed to the US to work in a children's summer camp. The intention was to work as a kitchen hand in a camp in New York state, but upon arrival he was a little dismayed to discover that all the campers had 'special needs'. He was dismayed further when they informed him that they had recruited too many kitchen staff and would he mind stepping in as a carer, as someone had not arrived. The idea of living, eating and sleeping with eight teenagers with varying degrees of learning disabilities for three months horrified Paul; however, as the alternative was to go home, he decided to give it go! Having enjoyed the most amazing summer he signed up for the following year. Intermittently he gained further care experience in the UK. Paul then went on to become a qualified learning disability nurse and enjoyed many years working in a variety of settings. He is now a lecturer in learning disability nursing. Paul's main interest, which is reflected in his practice, teaching and indeed the topic for the chapter in this publication, is very much those who have a learning disability and associated mental health problems.

Dr Malcolm Peter McIver, PhD, MA (Dist), BA (Hons), RNT, RCNT, PDN, Dip Nursing (Lon), RNMH, ENG

Currently teaching in the faculty of Health and Human Sciences at the University of Hertfordshire, Malcolm has lectured on legislation and the rights of people with a learning disability for many years in a number of universities across the UK, and as a visiting lecturer to the University of Washington.

Alan Randle, RNLD, MSc, Integrative Adult Therapist

Alan Randle is a Senior Lecturer at the University of Hertfordshire in Learning Disabilities (LD) and Counselling. He trained as a nurse for people with LD at North Warwickshire School of Nursing and subsequently qualified as a community nurse at Reading University. He further obtained an MSc in Learning Disabilities studies at Hull University. Alan became interested in psychotherapy and communication with people with learning disabilities and qualified as an Integrative Adult Psychotherapist. He has maintained his curiosity in these areas and has developed an MA is Psychotherapy and Disability. Alan maintains a private practice and also facilitates groups. He also provides supervision to therapists who facilitate groups for people with learning disabilities.

Tracey-Jo Simpson, RNLD, qualified lecturer in Further Education, External Examiner for City & Guilds

Tracey-Jo Simpson is a Registered Learning Disability Nurse and qualified lecturer in further education. Throughout her years working in the NHS she supported people within an assessment and treatment service, who had mental ill-health as well as a learning disability. Whilst in this service she was part of a pilot scheme which supported women who had a learning disability to receive cervical screening. Now a self-employed practitioner, her work is extremely varied and includes guest lecturing at the University of Hertfordshire, off-site Practice-Teaching students who are studying for the combined degree in Social Work and Learning Disability Nursing, running a range of workshops and being an external examiner for City & Guilds.

Jacky Vincent, Registered Nurse in Learning Disabilities (RNLD), BA (Hons) in Healthcare Care Management

Jacky has over 15 years' experience in learning disability nursing. For the past few years, Jacky has been working as a Senior Nurse for Hertfordshire County Council and Hertfordshire Partnership NHS Trust. She predominantly provides clinical leadership and advice to the Community Learning Disability Nurses across Hertfordshire, as well as leading on practice initiatives including Essence of Care.

Jacky is presently seconded as a job-share into the position of Lead Nurse for the Learning Disability Directorate, providing nursing leadership and professional advice for the nurses, ensuring that mechanisms are in place to support and facilitate staff in the delivery of safe and effective care.

Acknowledgements

We would like to thank all of our colleagues for their help, support, comments and suggestions.

Debra would particularly like to thank her husband and children for their continued support, encouragement and love.

Ian would like to thank his partner for all of his continued support and encouragement.

Introduction

People with learning disabilities are one of the most vulnerable groups in society (Department of Health 2001). This book aims to provide readers – those who provide or wish to provide health care and support for adults with learning disabilities – with a foundation for their interventions. Contributors to this text come from a variety of backgrounds – in clinical practice and the academic world. The contributors are dedicated to creating and maintaining a positive environment for all; they believe that each person with a learning disability is a unique being, with individual needs and ambitions; they also believe that people with learning disabilities can lead full and rewarding lives – indeed, many already do so. Each chapter sets out to reflect these hopes and aspirations.

It is acknowledged that there are some people with learning disabilities who are marginalised by society, and experience prejudice, bullying, insensitive care and discrimination. The effects of these can have a damaging impact on the individual (Department of Health 2001). The majority of people with learning disabilities want to live an 'ordinary' life, having the independence and choice to make decisions about their lives (King's Fund 1999). There may be those who cannot make the choice or decision themselves and the Mental Capacity Act 2005 sets out ways in which those who cannot make those decisions are protected (Department of Health 2005b). Caring for and supporting those who have a learning disability can be complex, but at the same time rewarding – contributing to the person's well-being can be very satisfying for all concerned.

We are resolute in the belief that people with a learning disability are worthy of the best possible care and support; for you to do this, it is vital that you have an insight into and understanding of the key issues that impinge on the person's life, both in the community and also in the various health and social care settings. Those people who have a learning disability and are supported effectively in the community can become full, participating members of the community. We encourage you to promote the possibilities associated with living with a learning disability, by providing innovative and creative approaches to care and support and by acting as a knowledgeable doer and, most importantly, an advocate. Partnership working is key to successful and client-centred care; it is essential if care and support are to be delivered in the most appropriate manner that you are encouraged to apply

Caring for People with Learning Disabilities. Edited by I. Peate and D. Fearns.
Copyright © 2006 by John Wiley & Sons, Ltd.

this approach to care delivery in the situations in which you are working. Stressing the importance of partnership working and acknowledging the benefits that this may bring the individual mean looking beyond a disease-oriented approach to one in which the patient is central. Such an approach is on a par with the current Government's desires to make available a health service that is designed around the patient instead of the service (Department of Health 2006).

Nursing students, those who are undertaking NVQ/SNVQ, Access to Nursing and Cadet nursing programmes of study, and those who are returning to practice will be the prime users of this text – however, not exclusively those cited. This is not a text that will provide you with a panacea for all of the needs of those who have a learning disability; it encourages the reader to identify further areas of importance that may not have been discussed here and to investigate further and deeper. Within the text, the terms 'nurse', 'student' and 'nursing' have been used. The terms and the philosophies applied in this book can be adapted to suit a number of health and social care workers at various levels and in a variety of settings in order to develop caring, informed skills.

The book utilises up-to-date information that the reader will need in order to begin to understand how to help, support and care for those individuals with learning disabilities in the institutional setting (e.g. the hospital) and in the community (e.g. the person's own home setting). The information is arranged in such a way that it reflects current health and social care practice in a user-friendly manner; furthermore, information is related to practice issues that may be encountered when working with people with a learning disability, their families and friends. We would not anticipate that the text be read from cover to cover in one sitting; rather, it can be used as a reference book (a resource, a reader), be it in the clinical setting, the classroom or your own home.

The text can be considered as a handbook or a manual that has an up-to-date evidence base; it is anticipated that it will challenge and encourage the reader to acquire a questioning approach to care provision, emphasising the important relationship between theory and practice. You may be studying at the moment; if this is the case, in order for you to get the most out of this book, you are encouraged to attend all of your classes associated with your current programme of study, and we would suggest that you use this text to supplement your current learning.

Most of the content relates and refers to some key health and social care documents, publications and statues that are used here to inform debate. One key government publication – *Valuing People: A New Strategy for Learning Disabilities for the 21st Century* (Department of Health 2001) – is central, explicitly or implicitly, to deliberations.

The wide-ranging aim is to facilitate understanding associated with essential aspects of care in an attempt to enhance safe and effective care, and to encourage and generate discussion. It is anticipated that the outcome will improve the quality of care provision that is underpinned by an informed knowledge base. This book is a fundamental text that can enhance personal and professional growth in relation to learning disability care.

CONTEMPORARY SOCIETY

It is estimated that there are over 800,000 people in the UK aged over 20 years who have a learning disability (Department of Health 2005a); putting this into context can help you to understand the needs of those whom you may need to provide care and support for, as well as the extent of the challenges. This number is expected to rise by 14 per cent to 900,000 by 2021. Furthermore, the number of those with severe learning disabilities may also rise by 1 per cent per year for the next 15 years (Department of Health 2005a).

KEY TERMS

The choice of terms used in this text is diverse. It is important to define terms from the beginning; different terms may mean different things to different people. There are a variety of terms that can be used to describe people with learning disabilities. The use of any term has the ability to label the person to whom the term is being applied. Labelling may lead to prejudice and discrimination, and can result in stigmatisation. Stigma is powerful and can have negative consequences for an individual's identity.

Often, the term 'patient' is used in healthcare settings. Not everyone supports its use, as it has passive connotations associated with it; it can also highlight the medical focus of the relationship between the person and the service. On occasions, 'client' is used; this has the ability to stress the professional nature of the relationship. More recently, the term 'expert' has been used, with the emphasis on a participative approach, acknowledging a person's capacity to work towards his/her own rehabilitation. Experts are seen to be equal partners with experts who provide care, such as a nurse or doctor. Not everyone is keen on the term 'service user' or 'user'. The term 'user' may also have negative connotations associated with it. It may be used to single out those who use illicit substances.

'Adults with a learning disability' is a term that has been used in the title of this text and also in this introductory aspect of the book. This is a broad definition, often used by various health and social care agencies. It has the potential to recognise that many people can and do have a learning disability, but they may not necessarily have an illness or a disease.

Various terms are used in this text with the aim of promoting the care and support of individuals with learning disabilities. The terms we have used address a wide range of experiences that may affect members of our society. In order to avoid stigma, prejudice and stereotyping, listen to and respect the terminology that is being used by those who are living with a learning disability.

The word 'carer' has been used on many occasions in this book. It is used to describe those who look after others, whether they be ill or healthy, or have a disability. 'Carer' has many interpretations and may refer to an employed healthcare provider or someone who provides care that is unpaid. It has been estimated that there are approximately 6 million unpaid carers in the United Kingdom (Carers UK 2005); this includes parents, grandparents and siblings who are looking after people with learning disabilities.

THE CHAPTERS

It is impossible to discuss all elements of health and social care related to the person with a learning disability. We have arranged the chapters in such a manner as to provide you with some insight into the intricacies associated with the care and support that may be required by an individual who has a learning disability. Primarily, we aim to provide you with the essence of care and a fundamental understanding of some of the issues that may impinge on a person's well-being.

Central to Chapter 1 is the importance of fostering good working relationships with adults who have learning disabilities. Key concepts such as person-centred planning will be considered and debated in detail, as well as the diversity of the varying needs of adults with learning disabilities. Approaches to care are examined.

Chapter 2 focuses on effective communication strategies that can be used for adults with learning disabilities; processes and forms of communication are outlined. The chapter makes clear how important it is to assess social functioning, as well as communication skills, when determining need. There are those individuals who have communication problems, as a result of which communication policies must be developed to disseminate information in accessible formats; some of these formats are outlined. In addition, there will be discussion concerning barriers to communication, including non-verbal communication processes.

Caring for and supporting the individual who presents with behaviours that may pose challenges are outlined in Chapter 3. There are various methods that may be used to support and manage a person with learning disabilities when their behaviour poses problems. Interventions will be examined and placed within the context of 'normalisation' principles underpinning learning disability care and provision. The chapter points out that over-reliance on psychotropic drugs can often result in poor outcomes as a consequence of their use. Management strategies will be discussed and outlined.

Chapter 4 provides the reader with an understanding of how to protect the 'vulnerable' adult who has learning disabilities from exploitation and abuse; protection is seen as paramount. This chapter will outline policies and procedures that are in place to ensure the protection of the 'vulnerable' learning disabled adult and identification of the 'vulnerable' adult 'at risk'. The chapter uses the *No Secrets* publication to demonstrate that there is no place to hide when it comes to exposing the abuse of vulnerable adults (Department of Health and Home Office 2000). The chapter draws upon the legal framework in place, identifying voluntary and statutory provision. Chapter 9 discusses the framework and other legal issues further.

The incidence and prevalence of mental ill health in adults with learning disabilities is higher than within the general population. In Chapter 5, vulnerability factors are discussed and highlighted, including how these may contribute to mental health difficulties. Issues around diagnosis and treatment are explored. The chapter emphasises the point that those who have a learning disability as well as a mental health illness should be able to access services and be treated in the same way as anybody else.

Chapter 6 focuses on the person with a learning disability who also has epilepsy. Epilepsy is defined and the categories of epilepsy outlined. The management of epilepsy will be examined and strategies discussed. The use of anti-epileptic drugs (AEDs) will be examined in the context of recently published National Institute for Health and Clinical Excellence (NICE) guidelines as well as the *National Service Framework for Long Term Conditions* (Department of Health 2005c).

Fulfilling the health potential of adults with learning disabilities is central to care; Chapter 7 discusses health promotion initiatives. These activities consider some of the special health needs of adults with learning disabilities and how they can be empowered to meet these needs. Discussion of opportunist health promotion and health promotion activities will be included; emphasis is placed on making health material accessible to those who have learning disabilities.

Since the text will consider a range of issues related to health and illness and the impact on adults with learning disabilities, Chapter 8 describes some biophysical aspects of anatomy and physiology, identifying how these may relate to specific syndromes, e.g. Down's syndrome. Fundamental aspects of the physical characteristics of Down's syndrome will be examined in relation to specific medical issues, such as heart and circulation, the digestive system, etc. This will be followed by discussion of potential difficulties that the adult with Down's syndrome may encounter, such as congenital heart defects and hypertension.

Caring for adults with learning disabilities will inevitably involve ethical, moral and legal issues. Chapter 4 has already begun to address these issues;

Chapter 9 continues to address other concerns, such as civil rights. Often, these issues are complex; this chapter highlights ethical theories and focuses on the legal ramifications in such a way that the reader is able to relate them to practice.

The final chapter addresses the rights of adults with learning disabilities to marry and have children; this is at the heart of *Valuing People* (Department of Health 2001). The number of people with learning disabilities who are forming relationships and having children has steadily increased over the last 20 years. This brings with it many challenges, hopes and aspirations. This chapter discusses anti-discriminatory practice, drawing on the discussions made in other chapters, supporting parents and examining practical aspects of inter-agency working that can support parents with learning disabilities, whilst being aware of issues of child protection and children 'at risk'.

We hope that by using this text to support your practice, you are able to advocate and support the person with a learning disability in a variety of settings. We are delighted that you have chosen to care for and support those who have learning disabilities and we are confident that you really will make a difference.

REFERENCES

Carers UK (2005) *A Manifesto for Carers*, London, Carers UK.

Department of Health (2001) *Valuing People: A New Strategy for Learning Disabilities for the 21st Century*, London, HMSO.

Department of Health (2005a) *Learning Disability Task Force: Annual Report 2004 – Challenging, Listening, Helping to Improve Lives*, London, Department of Health.

Department of Health (2005b) *Independence, Well-being and Choice: Our Vision for the Future of Social Care for Adults in England*, London, Department of Health.

Department of Health (2005c) *National Service Framework for Long Term Conditions*, London, Department of Health.

Department of Health (2006) *Our Health, Our Care, Our Say: A New Direction for Community Services*, London, Department of Health.

Department of Health and Home Office (2000) *No Secrets: Guidance on Developing and Implementing Multi-Agency Policies and Procedures to Protect Vulnerable Adults from Abuse*, London, Department of Health.

King's Fund (1999) *Learning Disabilities: From Care to Citizenship*, London, King's Fund.

1 Working with Adults with Learning Disabilities

JACKIE KELLY

KEY POINTS

- The definition of the term 'learning disability' has historical roots and, over time, the way in which the term has been defined has changed.
- Person-centred planning is central to the care of people with learning disabilities.
- Carers must be aware of and respect the values and rights of each individual.
- Fostering good working relationships with adults with learning disabilities and the employment of a variety of innovative communication and inter-personal skills are paramount in ensuring effective support.

INTRODUCTION

In this introductory chapter, the overarching focus will be to present a range of ideas designed to foster effective working relationships with adults with learning disabilities, their families and other people involved in their lives (Emerson et al. 2005). Some ideas introduced may be further developed in subsequent chapters of the text; these links will be noted, as appropriate.

Both the diversity of needs of people with learning disabilities and the importance of carers and teams being aware of this diversity of needs when working with and offering support to individuals will be key themes threaded through the following sections of this chapter.

In the first section, 'learning disability' will be defined and current philosophies of care and support for adults with learning disabilities will be explored. The key concept of person-centred planning as an approach to care will be addressed, emphasising the direction given by the government White Paper *Valuing People: A New Strategy for Learning Disability for the 21st Century* (Department of Health 2001a).

Caring for People with Learning Disabilities. Edited by I. Peate and D. Fearns.
Copyright © 2006 by John Wiley & Sons, Ltd.

In the second section, the importance of establishing, maintaining and ending therapeutic relationships with adults with learning disabilities will be discussed. It will also highlight the importance of carers being aware of values and rights issues for adults with learning disabilities.

In the third section, issues of diversity will be highlighted; in particular, cultural issues and issues for older adults with learning disabilities will be noted. Varying needs will be explored, considering issues relating to day-to-day care, housing, work opportunities and expressions of sexuality.

In the fourth section, the potential of a range of therapeutic care approaches, such as empowerment, advocacy and person-centred care, will be explored. The application of particular care approaches/interventions will be demonstrated, as well as how they might enable us to address identified needs for the adult with a learning disability.

The final section of the chapter will conclude the previous discussions.

DEFINING A LEARNING DISABILITY

Before discussing needs and support issues, it is important to try to define this group of people that we term as 'adults with learning disabilities'. On the surface, this may seem a simple task. However, reviewing the historical context of learning disability care reveals a variety of ways in which the term has been defined over time (Department of Health 2001a; Gates 2003; Grant et al. 2005; O'Hara & Sperlinger 1997).

In March 2001, the Government produced a White Paper entitled *Valuing People: A New Strategy for Learning Disability for the 21st Century* (Department of Health 2001a). Within this document, not only do they seek to define and identify this group of people with 'learning disability', but also attempt to provide policy guidance for staff and carers who work with and support adults with learning disabilities. This was the first White Paper produced in over a decade in relation to the care and support of adults with learning disabilities, and hence it has great influence in determining the approaches currently adopted in caring for and supporting adults and children with a learning disability.

Within the White Paper, a person is described as having a learning disability if they have:

'• A significantly reduced ability to understand new or complex information, to learn new skills (impaired intelligence), with;
• A reduced ability to cope independently (impaired social functioning);
• Which started before adulthood, with a lasting effect on development.'

(Department of Health 2001a, p. 14)

This definition has shaped this chapter. However, it must be acknowledged that there is an ongoing debate regarding what defines learning disability and the associated difficulties of labelling a group of people in the first place. Acknowledgement is given to the importance of such debate; however, this is not included in the remit of this chapter.

It is valuable to note the importance of language and the context of the environment within which you may be working.

The term 'learning difficulty' can be attributed different meanings. For example, a person who has dyslexia can be said to have a learning *difficulty* but not necessarily a learning *disability*. Also, within some work environments, particularly within social care settings, the term 'learning difficulty' is often taken to mean learning disability.

This is not designed to make life confusing! However, it highlights the importance of clarification and the difficulty in categorising a group of people under a particular label. Hence, you can see how the number of people within the population who have a learning disability can be difficult to determine.

Following the definition above, the government estimates that there are approximately 1.4 million people in England with a learning disability. There are about 210,000 with a severe learning disability requiring a high level of support, and about 1.2 million people with a mild/moderate learning disability, which means these people may live independently, with varying needs of support (Department of Health 2001a). This will be further discussed later in the chapter.

CARE PHILOSOPHIES

Historically, we have moved from a situation in which adults with learning disabilities were cared for within institutional settings, such as learning disability specialist hospitals, to people being cared for in the community (Gates 2003). Many adults with learning disabilities have been, and will continue to be, cared for at home. Our encounters with adults with learning disabilities as carers, support staff and students tend to focus on those people receiving a higher level of support within a variety of service contexts. You may find yourself working with people to support them within their own homes, as noted above, or complementing the care provided by family members. Other settings may include NHS services, such as assessment and treatment services; social care environments run by local authorities; or private and/or voluntary organisations such as Mencap.

We have moved away from a philosophy according to which the person with a learning disability was cared *for* to a situation in which we actively seek to work *with* the person, to enable him/her to develop a greater level of independence with meaningful power and control over the decisions taken within his/her life. To this end, an approach called 'person-centred planning' (PCP) currently influences how staff and carers plan and deliver support with individuals.

PERSON-CENTRED PLANNING

Until the 1950s, the idea that adults with learning disabilities' had unique individual needs and rights was unheard of. Since that time, significant conceptual ideas have influenced policy development and subsequently changed the way in which services are delivered for adults with learning disabilities. It is valuable to briefly explore the journey and progression of thinking that have moved ideas from this custodial climate to one of more personal power control and inclusion.

The development of the Human Rights movement in the 1960s, and the work of Goffman (1961) in relation to the injustices experienced by people living in large institutional settings, laid the ground for radical change in service delivery for people with learning disabilities.

Perhaps the most influential idea to emerge was introduced by Wolfensberger in Sweden in the 1970s. The principle of 'normalisation' sought to direct us to utilise our resources to provide services that ensured that adults with learning disabilities were enabled to experience the same opportunities as any other adult within their cultural context (Wolfensberger 1972). Wolfensberger further developed this idea to include the concept of socially valued roles for people with learning disabilities, aptly termed Social Role Valorisation (SRV) (Wolfensberger 1998). SRV emphasised the need for adults to be given opportunities to develop roles within society that were valued by others in that society, such as the opportunity to be in paid employment, to use local social/recreation facilities or to have the right to express their sexuality – in other words, to have their individuality recognised, valued and respected.

O'Brien and Tyne (1981, cited in Gates 2003) interpreted these concepts in the United Kingdom, developing five service accomplishments: community presence, choice, competence, community participation and respect. Many of the services still use adaptations of these accomplishments in setting their service aims and objectives.

The People First service user movement, developed in the 1980s, heralded the beginning of a real contribution by adults with learning disabilities in the planning and development of services provided to support their own needs. The NHS and Community Care Act 1990 saw the emphasis being based on community care, highlighting the rights of adults with learning disabilities to be active participating members of the community, living and working within that community.

Within the process of care delivery, this emphasis on adults with learning disabilities being allowed to exist and contribute as individual, valued human beings was expanded further through the development of Individual Programme Planning (IPP). IPP asserted that adults with learning disabilities had the right to be involved in the assessment, planning, delivery and evaluation of their care. Adults with learning disabilities and their families were encouraged to actively participate in their needs assessments, in planning and review meetings. Key worker systems were established to help demystify these processes for adults with learning disabilities and allow them to make a valued contribution to the multidisciplinary approach offered by IPP. This was a significant concept and worked well to enable adults to be included in their own care assessment, management and delivery.

Adopting a person-centred approach (PCA) embraces some of the ideas within IPP but takes the concept to a higher level, as it incorporates greater involvement and responsibility for adults with learning disabilities in the decisions made in their lives.

This PCA is the contemporary concept adopted by service commissioners and providers in outlining the context and manner in which care provision for adults with learning disabilities will be constructed and delivered in the twenty-first century. It is a change not only in the processes of how we assess needs and subsequently set objectives and deliver services, but is a whole shift in the value base of services – a new way of thinking – and, as such, has a huge impact on the way in which carers and other professionals will be trained and educated to support adults with learning disabilities.

Within the constructs of *Valuing People* (Department of Health 2001a), a PCA to planning care is defined as:

'A process for continual listening and learning focussing on what is important to someone now and in the future, and acting upon this alliance with their family and friends. The listening is used to understand a person's capacities and choices. Person centred planning is the basis for problem solving and negotiation to mobilise the necessary resources to pursue a person's aspirations. These resources may be obtained from someone's own network, service providers or from non-specialist and non-service sources.'

(Department of Health 2001b, p. 12)

This definition is a directive from the Government, outlining how they interpret this concept of *person centredness* and providing carers working in support of individuals with a framework enabling this concept to be turned into a reality.

Adopting a PCA creates vast opportunities and challenges in supporting adults with learning disabilities.

The emphasis is on power and control being taken away from the service providers and placed squarely with adults with learning disabilities and their families and support networks, and represents a radical change from previous care delivery models.

Previously, choice and empowerment were valued, but such choice existed within a 'set menu' of services from which adults with learning disabilities had to choose. They were asked to fit in to whatever was the most appropriate service to meet their needs.

A PCA through PCP sees adults with learning disabilities identifying their own needs with their families and personal support circle, in partnership with service providers. It requires service providers to look at using resources to meet these individual needs, rather than fitting people into existing services.

PCP allows adults with learning disabilities to aspire beyond their current worlds. It gives people the opportunity to have dreams for the future. It takes away the focus on skills and deficits in their abilities and embraces creativity and innovative opportunities denied to adults with learning disabilities until now.

Community learning disability nursing aims to include individuals in their planning meetings. However, frustrations can be experienced in the scope of this inclusion. Adults with learning disabilities are sometimes present at meetings but conversations may be taken over by some professionals with their own agendas when acting in the 'best interest' of the individual. A PCA means just that – the adult with a learning disability sets the agenda; meetings are not set at particular times, but occur when required. The agenda both for the meetings and for individual lifestyle planning is set, directed and controlled by the adult with a learning disability, his/her advocates and supporters:

> 'A person-centred approach to planning means that planning should start with the individual (not with services), and take account of their wishes and aspirations. Person-centred planning is a mechanism for reflecting the needs and preferences of a person with a learning disability and covers such issues as housing, education, employment and leisure.'
>
> (Department of Health 2001a, p. 49)

Smull (2004, cited in Grant et al. 2005) makes a poignant observation, demonstrating the need for care providers to change their attitudes. He talks about comfort rituals, noting that we would not deny ourselves a glass of wine for relaxation at the end of a 'bad' day, but would probably feel it was all the more reason to indulge in this comfort, whereas people with learning disabilities are often denied their comfort ritual if they have not been 'good', or have had a 'bad day'. This is a valid point in terms of care providers' controlling people's lives, and involves carers' having to change their attitudes and perceptions to give back that control to where it belongs – to the people themselves.

Criticism has suggested that a PCA is a concept that sounds ideal and forward-thinking; however, as with many well-intentioned concepts and ideas, it is open to interpretation. Hence, the true meaning and consequence of a PCA are still developing and we need to be conscious that the essence and original intentions of the approach are not lost. Other critics highlight the difficulties in service providers' responding to individual needs effectively in shifting resources to ensure that appropriate opportunities are available.

The reliance on unpaid carers and a circle of support for the person with a learning disability could exclude some adults with learning disabilities who, by the very nature of their needs and circumstances, may not have established trusted networks to support them. An example would be a person who has a high level of need with limited communication abilities and living in an institutional setting with little or no family contact. Such people will rely on paid professionals and carers to ensure that they have access to this approach to planning their lives (Grant et al. 2005).

As carers involved in supporting adults with learning disabilities, you need to ensure that you are equipped to provide appropriate support. Hence, you will need to be aware of PCP initiatives in the services that you will be working in:

> 'PCP may be best considered an evolutionary step in the long-standing trend towards the increasing individualisation of services.'
>
> (Emerson et al. 2005)

You will need to develop innovative communication and interpersonal skills and be imaginative, along with colleagues, advocates and family members, in exploring creative ways to ensure that adults with learning disabilities take control of their life planning. Communication and interpersonal issues will be further explored by Randle in Chapter 2 of this book; however, the following section will explore issues relating to the need for you as a carer or student to be aware of the importance of fostering good working relationships with adults with learning disabilities.

ESTABLISHING, MAINTAINING AND ENDING THERAPEUTIC RELATIONSHIPS

The process of, and considerations for, effective communication with adults with learning disabilities will be discussed in Chapter 2 ('Communication and Adults with Learning Disabilities'). This section will explore key considerations and reflect on establishing, maintaining and ending therapeutic relationships.

When thinking about our contact with another person, first impressions can be significant in setting the tone for building a rapport and relationship with that person in whatever context we encounter one another.

Reflecting my experience as a student nurse, contact with adults with learning disabilities prior to commencing the course related to working in a school for children with special educational needs and family contacts with individuals with mild learning disabilities and/or Down's syndrome. As a student, arriving in a long-stay hospital for adults, with a variety of needs relating to their learning disabilities, while walking along a corridor, a fellow student and I encountered a young man with what could be described as significant facial and physical characteristics associated with his disability. I later discovered that this was acrofacial dysostosis (ACD) Catania type – a rare autosomal syndrome (Jablonski 2005).

Greeting this man, my initial response was to feel empathy, and to honestly assume that he would have limited ability to respond. My fellow student reflected feeling quite disturbed by this man's appearance. At this point, he 'blew a raspberry', poked his tongue out and proceeded on his way, leaving us quite dumbfounded!

Later opportunities to interact with this man enabled us to see the 'man behind the mask', and discover who he was as a person. The lesson here in thinking about our work with adults with learning disabilities is to remember that, first and foremost, they are people. We need to be aware of our own experiences of interacting with people with learning disabilities. We need to adopt a questioning approach, increasing our knowledge, thus reducing the opportunity for us to make assumptions and judgements about people based purely on their appearance or diagnosis. We need to utilise support mechanisms to address our learning needs, such as through supervision and appraisal processes. This will enable us to ensure that our practice is based on an anti-discriminatory approach (ADP) and help us to develop a heightened sense of awareness of ADP issues within the work environment and wider society. In Chapter 9 of this book, McIver discusses legislation addressing issues relating to ADP and legal concerns.

In treating people as individuals, we need to acknowledge their disabilities and adapt our communication and interaction to ensure that the adults have every opportunity to engage with us, and demonstrate who they are as individuals. Often, adults with learning disabilities rely on others to interpret and convey their messages, leaving them vulnerable to misinterpretation and misrepresentation. As a student or paid/voluntary carer, you will often be in the position of trying to establish meaningful communication and interaction with adults whom you support. You will need to ensure that you have the appropriate skills to take on this responsibility.

Alongside this awareness of beginning interpersonal relationships with adults with learning disabilities, consideration needs to be given to how to maintain these relationships, using everyday opportunities to engage in valued conversation. Often, as carers, our interaction with people is associated with personal care (Ambalu, in O'Hara & Sperlinger 1997). The demands of time and perhaps staffing levels can limit opportunities; care must be taken to guard against this and to be conscious of developing opportunities for 'real' conversations. We need to accept and value times at which people may choose not to interact with us, hence supporting people to be assertive and enabled to indicate to carers when they wish to disengage or be left alone, which is equally important (Ferris-Taylor, in Gates 2003).

Often, carers can find themselves in a position of power. As outlined above, you may be asked to initiate contact and conversations, as adults with learning disabilities may be reluctant to do so, for a variety of reasons, such as difficulty experienced in the communication process, type of disability or their life experiences. The last point can relate to some of the negative experiences that adults with learning disabilities may have had in past interactions. Hence, gaining trust and building a relationship over a period of time are important considerations, not only in establishing and maintaining relationships, but also in thinking about endings. This is particularly pertinent for carers who may encounter people for a fixed period of time, within a practice placement, for example.

It is important to consider ending relationships. Very practical strategies can include openness with people with whom you are working about the length of time you will be there. Using innovative ways to represent this may also be helpful, perhaps through use of a pictorial chart or adapted calendar to 'mark off the days'. You also need to ensure that the learning opportunities with which you engage are realistic within the given timeframe. Link any activities undertaken with a permanent staff member, working alongside him/her to ensure that continuity for the person is maintained when you leave.

Such endings are vital, as people with learning disabilities are often in environments in which they are reliant upon paid carers; inevitably, staff change and move on, leaving the person to build new relationships with new carers. This pattern of continual change and loss can affect both the person's ability and his/her desire to interact. This is a very important factor to consider within an educational context in which we are continually moving in and out of people's lives.

Appreciating the diversity of needs of adults with learning disabilities and developing an appropriate range of skills to support these needs necessitate opportunities for students to work with people in varied settings, who may have a wide range of needs. We have a responsibility to guard against negative outcomes for learning-disabled adults engaging with students and other staff during these opportunities.

Further issues of diversity are considered within the subsequent chapters of this book. The next section of this chapter will explore considerations specifically relating to culture and issues for older people.

ISSUES OF DIVERSITY, CULTURE AND THE NEEDS OF OLDER PEOPLE WITH LEARNING DISABILITIES

'People with learning disabilities from minority ethnic communities are at particular risk of discrimination in gaining access to appropriate healthcare. . . . Staff who understand the values and concerns of minority ethnic communities and who can communicate effectively with them have an important role to play in ensuring that minority ethnic communities can access the healthcare they need.'

(Department of Health 2001a, pp. 62–3)

The Government clearly outlines the necessity to profile cultural considerations in *Valuing People* (Department of Health 2001a). It further commissioned a report, *Learning Difficulties and Ethnicity*, in 2001, to specifically explore the needs of black and minority ethnic communities.

Comment is often heard from individuals and their families stating that they are doubly discriminated against, both having a learning disability and coming from a black or minority ethnic community:

> 'The simultaneous disadvantage experienced by individuals in relation to race, disability and gender has been termed "double disadvantage" or "triple jeopardy" in some research studies (Baxter et al. 1990; Butt and Mirza 1996).'
>
> (Mir & Raghavan, cited in Grant et al. 2005)

When working with adults with learning disabilities, an obligation to provide culturally sensitive care is required. To do this, we have to develop our knowledge base and awareness of issues of diversity and how they impact on people within their current context.

Gender considerations, for example, need to be considered, as many supported living environments provide a service for both men and women. The staff complement within these establishments employs both men and women. However, in some Asian communities, such mixed-gender environments are at odds with cultural values and beliefs (Shah 1992). People with learning disabilities may be limited in their abilities to express themselves as cultural beings. The need to be informed in order to provide appropriate opportunities for this expression is paramount. Being familiar with cultural heritage, religious beliefs and value bases will enhance the ability to explore creative ways in which to ensure that these aspects of a person's life are highlighted.

The use of interpreters, for example, is a practical way of communicating with people for whom English is not their first language. However, this does not absolve you as a carer from increasing your awareness and appreciation of culturally specific issues for the people with whom you work. Assumptions that interpreters or people who share a common cultural heritage will work more effectively with a person with a learning disability may not always be valid or be the person's preferred option. Noting issues of diversity within black and ethnic minority communities themselves can identify conflicts where the life experience of the minority ethnic group carer may have little in common with the person with whom s/he is working. The key is partnership, working with individuals, families and other support networks, in line with the recommendations of PCP – ensuring that people with learning disabilities have access to information presented in a format that they can relate to. For example, using pictures to support the written word, supplementing written or pictorial information with personal contact and discussion, and ensuring that information is delivered in the appropriate language/dialect can all help to increase opportunities.

It is also important to be aware of the 'broader picture', as difficulties are not only related to language information or access barriers, but may also relate to a care system structured to fit within Western value structures, thus creating a mismatch with other cultures and belief systems (Payne 2005). The challenge is to ensure that care is delivered in a culturally sensitive, flexible and adaptable way in partnership with adults with learning disabilities.

The 'double' discrimination noted earlier also reverberates in thinking of the needs of older people with learning disabilities, who, in themselves, can be viewed as a further 'minority' sector within an already disadvantaged group of people. Older people within society as a whole have experienced discrimination in relation to lack of access to services or support, and in being devalued in terms of their contribution to society.

The life expectancy of adults with learning disabilities has increased, to be very much in line with their contemporaries (Bigby, in Grant et al. 2005). Their individual needs are directly related to their life experiences, just as they would be for anyone else. However, in exploring this, it becomes evident that life experiences of people with learning disabilities may differ from those of older people within the general population. This will influence their needs and the role that you will undertake in supporting them.

Deterioration in both physiological and mental health can be a feature of older age. Some conditions associated with age can be more prevalent for people with learning disabilities; adults with Down's syndrome, cardiovascular disease and problems with thyroid function, for example, have some potential physiological health implications, as well as a higher risk of early-onset dementia or Alzheimer's disease (Moss & Lee, in Thompson & Pickering 2001). As carers and students involved in supporting people, you need to be aware of this potential, and ensure that you are informed of the signs and symptoms to look for, and from whom to seek appropriate help and support for the individual.

There also appears to be an assumption in society that older people suddenly change their interests with the onset of progressing years; it is important, therefore, to safeguard older people's rights to participate in society from a person-centred perspective. This involves allowing them to make their choices and decisions, rather than assuming that particular activities will be of interest simply because the person is older. In doing this, attention needs to be given to ensure that appropriate resources are made available for individuals to continue to lead expressive lives, despite the onset of older age. Older people bring with them their vast knowledge and experience of life, and can be an invaluable source of information and support for others.

Student nurses have reflected their interest in talking to older people with learning disabilities who, having lived a significant portion of their lives in institutional settings, provide an invaluable insight into the changes and progression of services and the need for us to be vigilant in continuing such developments. Regardless of age or disability, the needs, wants, desires, dreams and expectations of each person must be considered on an individual basis. There is a variety of 'tools' which enable us to support adults with learning disabilities to take control of their own lives and ensure that they are fulfilled.

The next section of this chapter will explore the application of empowerment, advocacy and PCA to providing support to individuals and how these can enable adults with learning disabilities to experience opportunities for greater choice, expression of rights and participation in the planning of their own lives.

Case study

Jennifer Carter is a 20-year-old white woman who lives at home with her parents, Elisabeth and John, and her younger brother, Ben, aged 17 years.

Jennifer has a learning disability and epilepsy, although this is well controlled with medication.

Elisabeth and John describe themselves as caring but over-protective parents and have always been reluctant to allow Jennifer too much independence, as they are concerned for her safety.

Jennifer states that she has a good relationship with Ben, but is often angry with him and her parents, as Ben gets to go out freely whilst she feels curtailed by her parents and their concerns regarding her health issues.

Jennifer attends college three days a week and is undertaking a cookery course. She would like to get a job in the catering industry, and has recently seen an advert for a part-time job in the college cafeteria.

Jennifer has regular visits from a community learning disability nurse to monitor her epilepsy, as well as infrequent visits from a social worker when required. The social worker supported Jennifer to access the college.

Recently, at a review meeting, Jennifer asked the social worker whether she would help her to apply for a job. Elisabeth and John were surprised and a little angry with Jennifer, as she had not told her family that she wished to apply for the job and this was the first time they were aware of it.

John explained that Jennifer could not possibly hold down a job. Jennifer appeared frustrated and told her father that he was unfair, as Ben was able to do other things. Jennifer explained that she wished to leave home and lead her own life.

Jennifer's parents were hurt and surprised at this 'outburst'. However, the social worker explained that Jennifer had the right to express her needs and suggested that they arrange a PCP meeting to explore Jennifer's wishes. Her parents reluctantly agreed.

Prior to the meeting, the social worker and community nurse met with Jennifer to discuss her concerns and wishes, and seek her advice on how she would like the meeting to be conducted, where it should be held, who should be present and what the agenda for discussion should be. Jennifer was advised to have an independent advocate present at the meeting. It was explained that this could be a person that Jennifer knew or could be from one of the local advocacy support groups. Jennifer opted for an independent person and a meeting was arranged between Jennifer and Christine, from the local advocacy support group.

During the meeting, the family found it difficult to support some of Jennifer's wishes; however, Jennifer was clear that she wanted more independence. A person-centred plan was drawn up, identifying Jennifer's needs and wishes and noting her parents' concerns. Christine was able to provide support for Jennifer, which she found invaluable, as it had been difficult to challenge her parents, to whom she was so close.

Initially, Jennifer moved to an independent living situation, but found this too isolating. She moved back with her parents, but, six months later, Jennifer moved to a supported housing project, living independently with a 24-hour support worker contact system. This reassured her parents, and Jennifer was pleased with her newly found independence. She applied for the job, but was unsuccessful, but is hopeful that other opportunities will come up. She has joined a club and has made some new friends. Her parents are still concerned for Jennifer, but have realised that she needed to have more choice and control in her life. Her mother reflected that, surprisingly, this has been positive for them, as they feel less concern for the future as they grow older and may be in a position of being unable to care for Jennifer. Jennifer has maintained her links with Christine, and is now actively involved in the advocacy group herself, enabling other people with learning disabilities to be empowered to advocate on their own behalf and make choices in their lives.

Jennifer's situation could be described as having a 'happy ending'. However, if we consider this from a non-disabled person's viewpoint, a similar struggle may exist, but be accompanied by a sense of acceptance of the 'empty nest syndrome' (Seligman & Darling 1997). For many parents, having a child with a learning disability can be associated with concern about the future – what contribution will their child make, or be able to make, and who will care for him/her when they are unable to? A vast number of factors will influence this: degree of disability, family support mechanisms, and their own resilience. Often, parents struggle to obtain appropriate services to support their child and his/her needs. Such struggles and concerns can require a great deal of energy and time and be all-consuming. Though parents may wish for their child to be independent, the expectation can be changed and/or challenged by the child's disability needs.

Jennifer's parents may have wanted her to have independence but may have become used to being the focal carers. Jennifer continued to need her parents' care and support but also needed her own space and opportunity for self-expression.

It is important to ensure that cultural sensitivity is taken into account when considering independence or any other aspect of an individual's life; in some cultures, for example, adult children remaining in the parental home is accepted or, in some cases, expected, whether they have a disability or not (Seligman & Darling 1997).

It is also important to note that in the example above, Jennifer had the ability to live more independently and was able to verbally express her wishes and participate actively in her life development and choices. For people with more severe or profound disabilities, the choices may be different and family support maintained for much longer. Parents have reflected the difficulty in facing the future in 'handing over' care to someone else.

The concepts of empowerment and advocacy noted in the case study are equally applicable to all people, regardless of disability, yet the manner in which people are empowered or enabled to advocate for themselves will inevitably be influenced by their abilities. Empowerment principles argue that knowledge comes from individuals and we have to use their knowledge to enable them to live what *they* perceive as fulfilled lives (Payne 2005). Considering that many of the people with whom you may work will have been marginalised, discriminated against and/or devalued, it is vitally important that you respect the fact that their experience of their own lives makes them the experts; only *they* can fully understand their experiences and wishes, and you must respect, value and support this expert view. It is important to keep in mind that advocacy is a vehicle through which a person can be empowered.

CONCLUSION

This chapter began by defining 'learning disability' and highlighting the importance of carers developing their awareness of potentially labelling a group of people because they have a particular area of need, i.e. learning disabilities. The government White Paper *Valuing People: A New Strategy for Learning Disability for the 21st Century* (Department of Health 2001a) clearly sets the agenda for us, in offering appropriate and effective support for adults with learning disabilities in their everyday lives.

The PCA has ensured a shift in the value base and the way in which we think about care delivery for adults with learning disabilities. The emphasis is placed on power and control, resting squarely with the individuals themselves. As students and carers working with people with learning disabilities in a variety of contexts, we need to ensure that we are adequately equipped with knowledge, skills and information to enable people to lead fulfilled lives. Fostering good working relationships with adults with learning disabilities and utilising a variety of innovative communication and interpersonal skills to ensure effectiveness in support are advocated.

This engagement with adults with learning disabilities must include a core principle that they are people first, and assumptions and judgements may need to be challenged both within and by us and within the wider society within which we live and work. As students and carers, we are in a position of power, and need to ensure that that power base is shifted back to the adults with learning disabilities, enabling them to set the agenda for our relationships and interactions with them.

Cultural sensitivity, as well as gender and age considerations, must be evident within our working practice. This can be achieved with the application of a range of therapeutic approaches, such as empowerment, advocacy and person-centredness, enabling real power and control for the individual to be achieved.

The case study within this chapter seeks to highlight the value of a PCA in supporting a person with a learning disability. As students and carers, we need to adapt and change our attitudes, ideas and working practices to ensure that adults with learning disabilities are afforded real opportunities to advocate on their own behalf and thus be empowered to lead the lives of *their* choosing.

REFERENCES

Department of Health (2001a) *Valuing People: A New Strategy for Learning Disabilities for the 21st Century*, London, HMSO.

Department of Health (2001b) *National Service Framework for Mental Health*, London, HMSO.

Emerson, E., Routledge, M., Robertson, J., Anderson, H., McIntosh, B., Joyce, T., et al. (2005) *The Impact of Person Centred Planning on the Life Experiences of People with Learning Disabilities: Conclusions and Recommendations*, London, Department of Health.

Gates, B. E. (2003) *Learning Disabilities towards Inclusion*, Edinburgh, Churchill Livingstone.

Grant, G., Goward, P., Richardson, M. & Ramcharan, P. (2005) *Learning Disability: A Life Cycle Approach to Valuing People*, London, Oxford University Press.

Goffman, E. (1961) *Asylums*, London, Penguin Books.

Jablonski's Multiple Congenital Anomaly/Mental Retardation (MCA/MR) Syndromes Database (2005), available online at *www.nlm.nih.gov/cgi/jablonski/syndrome* (accessed 18/12/05).

Payne, M. (2005) *Modern Social Work Theory*, 3rd edn, Basingstoke, Palgrave Macmillan.

O'Hara, J. & Sperlinger, A. (1997) *Adults with Learning Disabilities: A Practical Approach for Health Professionals*, Chichester, J. Wiley & Sons.

Seligman, M. & Darling, R. (1997) *Ordinary Families, Special Children: A Systems Approach to Childhood Disability*, London, The Guildford Press.

Shah, R. (1992) *The Silent Minority: Children with Disabilities in Asian Families*, London, National Children's Bureau.

Thompson, J. & Pickering, S. (2001) *Meeting the Health Needs of People who Have a Learning Disability*, London, Bailliere Tindall.

Wolfensberger, W. (1972) *The Principle of Normalisation in Human Services*, Toronto, National Institute on Mental Retardation.

Wolfensberger, W. (1998) *A Brief Introduction to Social Role Valorisation: A High Order Concept for Addressing the Plight of Socially Devalued People, and for Structuring Human Services*, New York, Training Institute for Human Services Planning, Leadership and Change Agentry (Syracruse University).

2 Communication and Adults with Learning Disabilities

ALAN RANDLE

KEY POINTS

- 'Communication' is a difficult, if not impossible, concept to define.
- There are several factors that can enhance or hinder communication when communicating with adults with learning disabilities.
- Communication is a much broader issue than just talking or verbal speech.
- An awareness of anti-discriminatory issues with regards to communication can help to improve the process.

INTRODUCTION

The purpose of this chapter is to provide a fundamental understanding of some of the main issues concerning communicating with service users who have learning disabilities. Service users with learning disabilities are not all the same and may communicate in a variety of ways. Adults with learning disabilities are not a homogeneous group of people who all need to be treated in a similar fashion. 'Disabilities, just like abilities, occur on a continuum and it is just as unhelpful to put all disabled people in the same category as it is to classify all able bodied people as one' (Marks 1999, p. 121). Therefore, it is important to have an understanding of communication and the processes involved in order to discover how this will be beneficial when communicating with adults with learning disabilities, as their ability to communicate will vary in the same way as with anyone else.

This chapter is divided into several sections. The first section deals with what communication is. This section will provide a definition of 'communication' and outline one of the basic models of communication. 'Verbal and Non-Verbal Communication' forms the second section, which briefly explores descriptions of language and discusses in more detail non-verbal communication; this is sometimes called body language. The third section addresses

Caring for People with Learning Disabilities. Edited by I. Peate and D. Fearns.
Copyright © 2006 by John Wiley & Sons, Ltd.

'Factors Influencing Communication' and outlines some of the many factors that can cause difficulties when communicating or interacting with people with learning disabilities. The fundamental issue of 'Ending and Breaks in Communication/Therapeutic Relationships' is articulated in the fourth section. This section touches on the sensitivity required when finishing a communicative encounter with a service user in an appropriate manner. This leads on to the fifth section: 'Anti-Discriminatory Practice'. This section covers how communication can be discriminatory and considers how attempts should be made to be aware of this and address discrimination wherever possible.

DEFINING 'COMMUNICATION'

This aspect of the chapter will provide general definitions and explanations of what communication is. Within this section, there will be a description of a fundamental model of communication. This will be explored further where appropriate in the other sections, thus setting the scene.

The majority of work with adults with learning disabilities involves a considerable amount of communication in any given interaction. Therefore, it is important that an understanding of some of the main dynamics that take place during any communicative activity is gained.

Definitions of 'communication' generally describe it as a process between two or more people and that the transmission of a message occurs between the people interacting with one another. More complex definitions include aspects relating to the context within which the communication occurs and intentionality. However, a definition of 'communication' is required for the purposes of this chapter. Thompson (2003, p. 10) discusses communication in great detail and draws on Fiske's (1990, cited in Thompson 2003) definition of 'communication', which describes it as 'social interaction through messages'.

The 'social' aspect of this definition indicates that communication takes place within a shared context (Thompson 2003). Within a healthcare setting, communication would be regarded as a social event during the transmission of more formal information-giving messages. The act of passing on health information would require 'checking out' understanding of the material, thus making it more of a communal and shared process, even though there will possibly be an imbalance with regard to relationship, roles and knowledge. The 'interaction' component demonstrates that there is likely to be more than one person involved during any communication and that messages will be passed from one to another. This is often where it can be important to consider the environment or context. Communicating with someone in a formal setting will differ from an informal environment, although the message being communicated could be the same. The final elements of the definition 'through messages' illustrate the variety of ways in which information can be transmitted from one person to another. Messages can be conveyed or passed to others in many ways and the following list illustrates some of these. Messages, according to Fraser (1997), can be communicated through:

- the use of vocabulary and grammar
- sequencing
- proxemics
- emotional and mental state
- coherence
- sophistication of the messages being offered or understood.

All these areas are relevant to adults with learning disabilities. For example, the vocabulary used by adults with learning disabilities may provide an indication of their level of understanding, and communication with them can be adapted accordingly. Also, in terms of proxemics, adults with learning disabilities may be standing very close to the person speaking; this might also convey that they have a hearing difficulty and need to stand closer than what would be considered usual, to hear what is being communicated.

One very important factor that is not explicit within the above definition is the issue of intentionality of the messages being conveyed. When people are communicating or interacting, they are often doing so intentionally, i.e. they want to communicate with the other person. However, occasionally, messages may be passed on or communicated that were not intentionally meant to be. These more subtle messages may be sensed and perhaps understood. For example, someone may be talking very quickly and his/her voice may have a quavering quality to it. This person may be nervous and may be trying to disguise his/her feelings, perhaps trying not to intentionally communicate his/her anxiety. However, the person listening may notice these subtle messages and sense and understand that the person speaking is nervous about something. A key skill in this respect is to decide whether it is important to attempt to address the unintended message or not. Sometimes, it may help to mention that something else is also being communicated. However, it can also make another person feel misunderstood or even persecuted. No two situations are ever likely to be exactly the same; therefore, each time an unintentional message is being 'read' or noticed as such, it will need to be considered, depending on the circumstances, as to whether it is addressed or not. This is when it is important to consider the environment or context, as mentioned above. The skill here is to think, 'Is the setting influencing what is being communicated?' and 'Is it relevant to mention it, or not?'

Understanding and misunderstanding are also important areas to consider alongside intentionality. These areas are sometimes discussed in terms of 'meaning' (Thompson 2003; Trevithick 2000). Sometimes, what is being communicated between two or more people is not always clearly understood and

Sender	→	Message/noise	→	Receiver

Figure 2.1. Shannon and Weaver's (1949) model

may even be misunderstood. This is not necessarily a bad thing, as long as there is sufficient safety for the people involved to express that they do not understand, or to explain that they have misunderstood some part of the communication. This misunderstanding was not intentional; however, it may still have occurred. It is important, therefore, to communicate clearly and effectively as well as checking out that communication has been received and understood as it was intended (Department of Health 2003).

Communication is complex; so, too, is any definition of the term. Fiske's (1990) definition of 'communication', cited in Thompson (2003), suggests that communication is social interaction through intentional and unintentional messages. You are encouraged to question and debate this definition amongst yourselves, your colleagues and peers. It is imperative to consider how these messages are transmitted from one of the communicators to the other.

The process model of communication is one of the simplest models that will provide a good grasp of how messages are sent and received by two or more parties. Thompson (2003) acknowledges Shannon and Weaver's (1949) model as the classic model. This fundamental model is illustrated above (see Figure 2.1).

The sender or transmitter is the person who starts or initiates the communicative process, by sending a message. S/he sends the message to someone – the receiver. The message is transmitted between the two parties. However, many factors can influence this process and the 'noise' element indicates any aspect that could affect the message being sent and received (Lerner 2003). These will be discussed in more detail in the third section, below. What is important to remember here is the fact that you will not only be a sender of messages; you will also be a receiver of messages initiated by someone else. Adults with learning disabilities may not always initiate communication in familiar ways. The skill here is to observe, be aware of and sensitive to any communicative cues or endeavours made by the people whom you are working with (Fraser 1997). The following section will continue to discuss some aspects related to observational skills when communicating, i.e. noticing non-verbal communicative messages.

VERBAL AND NON-VERBAL COMMUNICATION

The importance of verbal and non-verbal communication will be explored here. There will also be an explanation of language. However, the emphasis within this section will be with regard to non-verbal communication and adults with significant disabilities, i.e. the importance of 'levelling' when working with adults who use wheelchairs and listening (observationally) with the eyes as well as the ears. This is often referred to as 'active listening' (Thompson 2003). This section aims to highlight that communication is much broader than just talking or verbal speech.

It is important to acknowledge that communication is both verbal (language) and non-verbal (body language). To proceed with our discussion about these issues, we need first to define 'language':

'Language can be defined as the use of an organised system of codes'.

(McLaughlin 1998)

This code is a system of rules for arranging random symbols in an ordered and recognised manner that enables someone who understands the code to draw out the meaning of the code. If the arbitrary codes of language are not produced in the order familiar between the people interacting, understanding and communication are inhibited. For example, if some of the random symbols contained within the alphabet were presented in the manner of 'nruFtireu', you may be able to recognise the individual symbols but they would not be in an order that you are familiar with. However, if they were rearranged to 'Furniture', you would recognise the symbols and the order. This is because you and I have a shared understanding of the code. Therefore, language can be described as an organised system of codes, used by humans to communicate. There are inherent difficulties with the issues contained within the concept of language and adults with learning disabilities, such as basic understanding, the use of language and the difference between vocalisations and verbal language – these will have meaning for individuals. However, the above information about language is only a brief summary of a vast area of study; we need to move on and define non-verbal communication and its importance for adults with learning disabilities.

Very broadly, non-verbal communication can be described as any use of communication that does not involve or excludes speech. More commonly, non-verbal communication is often referred to as body language. This simple definition can be broken down into separate components that make up non-verbal communication. These are what are known as proxemics and kinesics (Lishman 1994). Proxemics includes the distance and closeness that individuals prefer to be to one another. Kinesics involves the movements, gestures, expression and eye contact (Kadushin & Kadushin 1997).

There are several skills that need to be developed when considering non-verbal forms of communication. The main one is learning to notice them in the first instance. Adults with learning disabilities may be unable to complete the full range of non-verbal activities to express themselves in a manner that is always familiar or perceived as correct. A very basic example would be someone who uses a wheelchair that is manoeuvred by care staff. In terms of proxemics, she or he would not be in a position to move further away or nearer to someone if she or he so wished. Imagine being positioned near to someone whom you would have preferred not to be close to. Also, consider being positioned far away from a friend whom you wanted to be closer to and were powerless to change your position. This could be made worse if you were also unable to communicate this desire to someone. These issues need to be considered sensitively.

On a more complex level, adults who have learning and physical disabilities may be further restricted in their expression of non-verbal communication. Literally, their physical disabilities would prevent them from being able to carry out certain gestures. For example, pay attention the next time you wish to fold your arms across your chest to protect yourself, defend yourself or just keep yourself warm on a cold day. Adults with learning disabilities and physical disabilities would be unable to do this if, for example, their physical disability involved limited arm movement. Therefore, they may not only have difficulty defending themselves if they felt the need to, but they may not even be able to communicate that they are feeling cold.

You should aim to be observant to indirect or minute non-verbal communication; this is sometimes referred to as 'listening' with your eyes as well as your ears. Those with limited arm movement, for example, who wished to express that they were feeling self-conscious or vulnerable may execute some non-verbal communicative gesture in an almost unnoticeable manner. They may turn their bodies very slightly – if possible, looking in the other direction or away from the person they were communicating with, or close their eyes. There is a danger with this approach. You may begin to develop the tendency to notice every little gesture that people make when you are communicating with them. Although, this is a good skill to develop, all non-verbal communication does not have to be commented upon and interpreted to mean something. This could lead to someone feeling exposed, misunderstood and persecuted. The skill that needs to be developed is to notice the non-verbal communication in relation to the context of the interaction or conversation and the surrounding environment.

Much of the psychological (Gross 2001) material regarding non-verbal communication highlights that approximately two-thirds of information is passed between people interacting on a non-verbal level. The other third would account for the verbal message being sent. Some adults with learning disabilities may rely more on non-verbal means of communicating. Therefore, your distance and gestures will also be important. If you are standing above or higher than someone who uses a wheelchair, you may miss important information that is being expressed non-verbally (Hartland-Rowe 2004). It is, therefore, important that you maintain an appropriate level in order that you are able to observe these communications. This is sometimes referred to as 'appropriate levelling'. You need to move, sit next to, kneel or crouch in order that the person has a better chance of communicating with you, as she or he is unable to move up to meet you at your height, position or level. In addition, it is important that you do not make assumptions about your understanding of someone's non-verbal communication. It can provide you with further information about what an individual may be conveying. However, you need to also be open to the fact that you may get it wrong and you may misunderstand something that was being expressed in a non-verbal manner. The value of this discussion on non-verbal communication highlights for us that non-verbal communication has a function and that it is important to always consider that individuals may be attempting to communicate something about themselves to us as well as wishing to communicate with us (Stenfert-Kroese et al. 1997). For example, service users with learning disabilities may become frustrated that you are misunderstanding what they are communicating and may become angry and upset. Behaviour that can be described as challenging is sometimes a form of non-verbal communication and expression and also has a function for the individual; these issues will now be explored in the next section.

FACTORS INFLUENCING COMMUNICATION

There is a multitude of factors that influence communication between practitioners and service users. This section will focus on some of these barriers. Adults who may exhibit behaviour that could be described as challenging will provide the clinical example here, as many challenging behaviours can be seen as a method of communication, and attempts should be made to understand these very important messages. The labelling of someone with challenging behaviour may induce fear and create a cyclical pattern of communication and contact being avoided with people who have idiosyncratic ways of communicating. The main factor that will be addressed is that of 'attitude' – not only the attitude of the service user, but more so the attitude of the practitioner. Attitude can be conveyed through tone of voice and touch.

The beginning of this chapter outlined one of the basic models of communication, i.e. there is a sender who initiates communication, the message being sent and a receiver of the communicated message. There are many factors that can influence this process; some of them will be considered here. The list below illustrates some of the possible factors that can affect any communicative encounter:

- personality
- mental state
- culture
- levels – of communication and understanding
- environment/context
- power imbalance/dynamics

- gender
- language – difference and use, e.g. jargon
- previous knowledge/experience
- attitude
- intentionality/perception – meaning
- non-verbal communication.

The above list is by no means exhaustive and we have considered some of the areas in the preceding material. There is insufficient space to address all these important factors. However, during the following discussion, some of the factors will be combined, such as mental state and attitude. One very important aspect that needs to be taken seriously into account when considering these factors is that they do not only affect communication from the service user's perspective, but they will also affect us and will influence how we communicate with people. The important component here is with regards to the encoded message produced by the sender and the decoding process required of the receiver of the message (Lerner 2003). For example, if service users were asked before an interview how they were feeling, they may give a brief social response and merely say 'Fine, thanks', using a rather sharp tone in their voices. However, you may observe that they were wringing their hands and pacing the floor (non-verbal cue), indicating that they were perhaps feeling a little nervous or anxious. Therefore, the encoded message of 'Fine, thanks' (verbal) would have been accompanied by the non-verbal cues and the underlying message might have been 'I don't feel like talking right now'. You may have picked up on all these cues that were implicit in the message and decoded the message appropriately and decided not to take the conversation any further. In this instance, their anxiety or mental state influenced the overall communication encounter.

However, communication does not always go so smoothly, particularly with adults with learning disabilities. McKenzie (2001) considered communication with adults with learning disabilities and compared their recognition of emotional states in themselves and in other people. Adults with learning disabilities may not recognise feelings or emotional states within themselves or others. 'Worry' is one of the most difficult feelings to recognise, as 'worry' could be taken to mean nervousness or anxiety, for example. Therefore, when people with learning disabilities feel anxious, they may exhibit challenging behaviour or even some other emotional state. Stenfert-Kroese et al. (1997) discuss personal meaning and behavioural issues, and note that:

'... professionals who work with people with learning disabilities sometimes describe the behaviours of their clients in a seemingly objective but meaningless way (e.g. attention seeking) rather than specifying the possible motivation or emotion driving that behaviour (e.g. wanting to make more friends or feeling bored or lonely), thus ignoring the meaning of the behaviour and labelling a person's wish for human contact in a negative way.'

(Stenfert-Kroese et al. 1997, p. 3)

The skill that the practitioner requires is to consider what is going on for the service users and what is happening around them. This includes your influence and how you might be affecting the communicative encounter. McKenzie's (2001) work also identified that photographs that included contextual information assisted adults with learning disabilities in choosing emotional states more correctly rather than pure line drawings. This therefore makes it important for us as practitioners to consider what is happening around a service user, rather than only taking into account what is immediately taking place, or the task (McKenzie 2001).

Challenging behaviours may take various forms and have a variety of meanings (Hodges 2003) (in Chapter 3 of this book, Joannides discusses the issue of challenging behaviour further). In addition, the person may prevent the very thing that is wanted or wished for, i.e. communication. For example, some challenging behaviour may push people away from them when what is longed for are understanding, contact and communication. Hodges (2003) provides us with some simple guidance when considering individual service users' behaviours. She suggests that 'Having behaviour understood is essential for the mental health of the client' (Hodges 2003, p. 96). She continues by outlining that practitioners may avoid interacting or engaging with individuals who exhibit challenging behaviour due to the difficulties associated with not knowing what is being communicated and this may be awkward or uncomfortable for the practitioner. Hodges (2003) also acknowledges that this is often unintentional on the part of the staff. Therefore, the skill required here is to take the risk and try to understand what is being communicated, even if we find this difficult. Service users who are trying to communicate something by exhibiting challenging behaviour may not respond in the way that would be considered as most appropriate when someone is trying to help and understand them. However, the effort that staff put into trying to understand these service users is likely to be well received on some level by them.

From a person-centred perspective, Pörtner (2001, p. 11) offers some guidance for us to consider here. She suggests that we do not always succeed in decoding service users' ways of expressing themselves, but that we need to take it seriously and to hold on to the fact that the expression has meaning for the service users.

The issue of the care environment and challenging behaviour has been acknowledged by Kevan (2003). This work highlights an essential factor when considering communication with adults with learning disabilities who can be described as challenging. Kevan (2003) draws our attention not only to the expressive communication of behaviour, but more importantly to the receptive difficulties that adults with learning disabilities may encounter. Returning briefly to our basic model of communication, i.e. sender – message – receiver, the receptive aspect is linked with the receiving of the message. Therefore, service users may not have received the message you sent due to their inability to decode the message accurately because of their limited cognitive abilities. Therefore, it is important to know the abilities of service users in order to ensure that your communication matches their abilities. In addition, adults with learning disabilities may miss important information if there are other distractions surrounding them. Also, they may not be able to track a complicated conversation and process the information quickly enough to contribute at the most appropriate moment (Fraser 1997). Taking these factors into consideration may minimise the chances of an episode of challenging behaviour's taking place.

One particular area that may create a potential situation for challenging behaviour to occur is the loss of an important relationship. Service users often have limited social contact with others and build friendships with care staff. The ending of a shift or, more importantly, when a member of staff leaves a care service means that it is vital to end and finish any relationships that have been established appropriately and sensitively (Mattison & Pistrang 2000).

ENDINGS AND BREAKS IN COMMUNICATION/ THERAPEUTIC RELATIONSHIPS

Unintentionally, communication with service users is perhaps not always ended or finished appropriately, such as walking away from service users without informing them of the reason behind this act, which might be as simple as forgetting to collect or bring something that is required for an activity, but was not communicated to the service users. You may know the exact reason for leaving, even if only briefly, but may have unintentionally not communicated this to the service users. They then may experience this as a break in the communication or activity, which may affect their interactions with you when you return. (This issue of communication could be considered from an attachment theory perspective.) Although these breaks in communication are important, they can be easily rectified; Fraser (1997) mentions this in terms of repair. The emphasis within this section will be on ending or finishing therapeutic work/communication with a service user. This is particularly important for students who may be introduced to service users, engage with them during a piece of work and leave at the end of the placement period. It is extremely important to finish, end and 'say goodbye' in a meaningful manner (Mattison & Pistrang 2000).

All of our interventions with adults with learning disabilities, or any other service user group, have a beginning, a middle and an end (Trevithick 2000).

Adults with learning disabilities may not always pick up on cues that indicate that a period of being engaged with someone has ended and Trevithick (2000) highlights that this may be experienced in an abrupt fashion. This may be partly due to the issues relating to pace and understanding. In a world in which the pace of life is based on what is considered as 'normal', adults with learning disabilities may experience being left behind (Pörtner 2001). Some of these issues have been briefly discussed above. The immensely valuable contribution made to the learning disability field by Mattison and Pistrang (2000, 2004) cannot go without mention in this section. Their study not only considered the views of staff members and their thoughts and feelings about disengaging with service users, but also provided us with a moving insight into how adults with learning disabilities feel about how the endings of relationships with staff are handled and dealt with. They discuss the limited literature within this area in a succinct manner and provide us with a clear and balanced view of the importance of ending therapeutic encounters in a sensitive and meaningful manner.

Mattison and Pistrang (2000) highlight how adults with learning disabilities have limited social networks and may rely on staff members for friendship, including emotional support, and, due to the nature of some disabilities (i.e. additional physical disabilities) and service support (e.g. shift patterns and staffing ratios), there may be difficulties in enabling service users to build other socially supportive networks. They go on to discuss in detail how service users may then feel the trauma of the loss of these significant relationships which were not ended in the most appropriate manner and that due to limited means of expression, this could lead to exaggerated behavioural issues, including withdrawal rather than more overt behavioural expressions of their upset, i.e. exhibiting challenging behaviour. Therefore, it is important to consider how any therapeutic intervention is commenced, worked through and processed, and ended. Two main skills are identified as important to take into account when ending a therapeutic relationship/encounter: to have some awareness of how service users with learning disabilities may respond to the ending of a therapeutic relationship or a communicative encounter, and to be able to help service users name and express their feelings (Mattison & Pistrang 2000). Whilst these authors do discuss more profound and significant losses overall, it is nonetheless important for us to consider these issues in relation to ending communication appropriately with service users. Fortunately, Mattison and Pistrang (2000) draw attention to the communication issues in relation to the above. Outlining that type and severity of the learning disability will call upon practitioners' skills in recognising how the service user's feelings are expressed and the skills required to assist with this process. This is explored further in their work, clearly suggesting that as staff members, we should not underestimate the impact that we have on service users. Knowing when to mention the ending to service users was also examined and the importance of preparation is indicated – some service users may have experienced the ending as more abrupt due to their disabilities; they may need the message repeated and reinforced (Emerson 1977, cited in Mattison & Pistrang 2000, 2004). The skill required here is at least to be aware when you are leaving, finishing or ending a communicative encounter with people with learning disabilities and to inform them as best you possibly can. Jackson and Jackson (1999) offer one possible alternative way of communicating with adults with limited abilities. They have produced a small piece of work demonstrating how they utilised photographs to help adults with learning disabilities communicate issues related to endings and losses.

ANTI-DISCRIMINATORY PRACTICE

Carers and students need to have a raised awareness of anti-discriminatory issues with regards to communication. This chapter started by outlining a basic model of communication and proceeded to explain the difficulties that may be encountered when interacting and communicating with adults with learning disabilities.

There are also other influencing factors that could affect any communication with an adult with a learning disability from a discriminatory perspective. A cultural difference may be that the service user and the practitioner are from different cultural backgrounds and that they may not have a thorough understanding of each other's cultural considerations. There could be a misunderstanding in relation to non-verbal communication, as discussed previously, such as eye contact, personal space (proxemics) and touch (Ferris-Taylor 2004). Verbal communication may be impeded by dialects and by the fact that individual members of staff may use words in different ways (Thompson 2003). These are very important issues to consider, particularly if the service user is also significantly learning disabled and has very limited communication abilities. The Department of Health (2001) report on *Learning Difficulties and Ethnicity* cautions us on broader issues relating to ethnicity and service provision which can be interpreted on an individual level. We need to be aware that individual service users may not be able to communicate their needs associated with their ethnicity. However, they may be in the 'most need'.

Whilst these issues are very important, there are much more subtle ways in which adults with learning disabilities can experience discrimination when communication or interaction is taking place. The words used to communicate and the speed or pace at which communication is delivered are two very powerful ways in which people with learning disabilities can be discriminated against. Developmentally, from the outset, adults with learning disabilities may have moved though the communication milestones at a slower rate

(Cuskelly et al. 2002; Fraser 1997; Graves 2000) than those without a learning disability. This is an indication that an individual with a learning disability may not have as extensive a range of words or vocabulary as someone of a similar age might have. This has been described and discussed in terms of a 'core' vocabulary and research has identified that adults with learning disabilities have a limited core vocabulary (Graves 2000). Therefore, if a carer expects or overestimates someone's receptive skill (Kevan 2003) and believes she or he *should* understand something, this is indirect discrimination. The skill here is to attempt to use simpler, easier and uncomplicated sentences to communicate. It is discriminatory to use very sophisticated words that people are unlikely to be able to comprehend. Perhaps use language that is more obvious to the situation or utilise the use of what are known as objects of reference. Broadly, 'objects of reference are used alongside other means of communication such as natural gestures and/or pictures' (Park 1995, p. 41 and Kevan 2003). Park (1995) also suggests that they are considered as 'bridges' that assist communication. A natural gesture might be miming drinking when asking someone if they would like a drink. Pictures can also provide more information. For example, a photograph of a local café that is familiar to the service user would offer assistance in helping an individual to understand that you might be suggesting having a drink at the café. Including other objects of reference such as the service user's coat will provide clues for the service user about what is being communicated. Offering these in the order in which they will happen may also be beneficial. Staff members need to use objects of reference for individual service users in a consistent fashion otherwise they could become confusing for a particular service user and will not assist communication.

In general use words and language are often spoken at some considerable speed. This can add to difficulties experienced if someone is trying to understand or decode the first word in any given sentence. Above, we discussed, briefly, Pörtner's (2001) thoughts about 'pace'. These issues are very relevant here. However, Cuskelly et al. (2002, p. 44) identify studies that have considered that adults with learning disabilities, specifically those with Down's syndrome, 'experience the power of communicating a message earlier than their speech difficulties will allow'. Therefore, what we need to consider here is the issue of time and timing. We need to allow service users time to respond to our requests or communications and it would be considered discriminatory to rush someone to respond at our pace. We need to allow more time for service users with limited cognitive abilities to process the information and respond at their own speed. The danger here could be that if service users were not given enough time to respond, they may eventually give up trying to communicate. Communicating with service users with learning disabilities at speed, at a level that they do not understand and in an overly sophisticated manner is discriminatory. This does not indicate that they need to be patronised. Taking someone's pace, understanding and abilities into consideration is being sensitive to their needs and is an endeavour to negotiate and interact with someone in an inclusive manner (Cuskelly et al. 2002).

These factors may also affect the ways in which service users and staff communicate with one another and may implicitly be discriminatory. Having an awareness of some of these factors will enhance communication endeavours with service users. These may not be able to be addressed in every circumstance. However, your attempts to understand and address any discrimination with regards to service users will be seen as good anti-discriminatory practice.

CONCLUSION

This chapter has aimed to articulate some of the difficulties related to communicating with adults with learning disabilities. Definitions of 'communication' were coupled with the basic process of communication, i.e. sender–message–receiver. Language and non-verbal communication were presented, highlighting the importance of noticing non-verbal communicative attempts made by adults with learning disabilities. However, the skill is knowing when and how to use this information to improve communication. The third section covered some of the many factors that can influence communication; one of the main ones discussed was emotional states. The importance of sensitively ending communications with adults with learning disabilities was highlighted. This is pertinent not only when ending what might be considered an insignificant interaction, but also when ending major therapeutic relationships. Finally, the chapter briefly explored some anti-discriminatory issues.

REFERENCES

Cuskelly, M., Jobling, A. & Buckley, S. (2002) *Down's Syndrome Across the Life Span*, London, Whurr Publishers.

Department of Health (2001) *Learning Difficulties and Ethnicity*, London, Department of Health.

Department of Health (2003) *Statement of Guiding Principles Relating to the Commissioning and Provision of Communication Skills in Pre-registration and Undergraduate Education for Healthcare Professionals*, London, Department of Health.

Ferris-Taylor, R. (2004) 'Communication: Helping People Achieve Independence and Wellbeing', in B. Gates (ed.), *Learning Disabilities*, 4th edn, London, Churchill Livingstone.

Fraser, B. (1997) 'Communicating with People with Learning Disabilities', in O. Russell (ed.), *Seminars in the Psychiatry of Learning Disabilities*, London, Gaskell.

Graves, J. (2000) 'Vocabulary Needs in Augmentative and Alternative Communication: A Sample of Conversational Topics Between Staff Providing Services to Adults with Learning Disabilities and their Service Users', *British Journal of Learning Disabilities*, **28**: 113–19.

Gross, R. D. (2001) *Psychology: The Science of Mind and Human Behaviour*, 4th edn, London, Hodder & Stoughton.

Hartland-Rowe, L. (2004) 'An Exploration of Severe Learning Disability in Adults and the Study of Early Interaction', in D. Simpson & L. Miller (eds), *Unexpected Gains: Psychotherapy with People with Learning Disabilities*, London, Karnac.

Hodges, S. (2003) *Counselling Adults with Learning Disabilities*, Basingstoke, Palgrave Macmillan.

Jackson, E. & Jackson, N. (1999) *Learning Disability in Focus: The Use of Photography in the Care of People with a Learning Disability*, London, Jessica Kingsley Publishers.

Kadushin, A. & Kadushin, G. (1997) *The Social Work Interview*, New York, Guilford Press.

Kevan, F. (2003) 'Challenging Behaviour and Communication Difficulties', *British Journal of Learning Disabilities*, **31**: 75–80.

Lerner, J. W. (2003) *Learning Disabilities: Theories, Diagnosis, and Teaching Strategies*, 9th edn, Boston, Houghton Mifflin Company.

Lishman, J. (1994) *Communication in Social Work*, Basingstoke, Macmillan.

Marks, D. (1999) *Disability: Controversial Debates and Psychosocial Perspectives*, London, Routledge.

Mattison, V. & Pistrang, N. (2000) *Saying Goodbye: When Keyworker Relationships End*, London, Free Association Books.

Mattison, V. & Pistrang, N. (2004) 'The Endings of Relationships between People with Learning Disabilities and their Keyworkers', in D. Simpson & L. Miller (eds), *Unexpected Gains: Psychotherapy with People with Learning Disabilities*, London, Karnac.

McKenzie, K. (2001) 'A Picture of Happiness', *Learning Disability Practice*, **4**(1): 26–9.

McLaughlin, S. (1998) *Introduction to Language Development*, London, Singular Publishing Company.

Park, K. (1995) 'Using Objects of Reference: A Review of the Literature', *European Journal of Special Needs Education*, **10**(1): 40–6.

Pörtner, M. (2001) *Trust and Understanding: The Person centred Approach to Everyday Care for People with Special Needs*, Ross-on-Wye, PCCS Books.

Shannon, C. E. & Weaver, W. (1949) *The mathematical theory of communication*. Urbana: University of Illinois Press.

Stenfert-Kroese, B., Dagnan, D. & Loumidis, K. (1997) *Cognitive Behavioural Therapy for People with Learning Disabilities*, London, Brunner-Routledge.

Thompson, N. (2003) *Communication and language: A Handbook of Theory and Practice*, Basingstoke, Palgrave Macmillan.

Trevithick, P. (2000) *Social Work Skills: A Practice Handbook*, Buckingham, Open University Press.

3 The Importance of Managing Behaviours which Pose Challenges

COSTAS JOANNIDES

KEY POINTS

- 'Challenging behaviour' is a complex term to define and understand; it is a term that is used often and can lead to prejudgements and stigmatisation.
- Challenging behaviour is functional; it may be an indication of physical discomfort, pain, emotional distress, mental illness or conflicts in the person's environment.
- A person's behaviour will be defined as challenging when it is judged by another to be socially unacceptable and when it evokes significant negative emotional responses in the other.
- Long-term, effective support for carers working with adults with learning disabilities with challenging behaviour is essential, as working in these situations is often stressful and difficult.

INTRODUCTION

This chapter will address issues centred on supporting and caring for adults with learning disabilities whose behaviours may pose problems. Management and care strategies will be discussed and outlined, and interventions will be examined and placed within the context of 'normalisation' principles underpinning learning disability care and provision. The overall aim of this chapter is to explore the issue of the phenomenon commonly described as 'challenging behaviour'. An explanation will be sought concerning assumptions, such as 'Is challenging behaviour an innate part of an individual's character or person, or is it a socially constructed product which one can assume can be deconstructed by creative strategies?'

Challenging behaviour is a label – in a field in which there are already too many. Carers and services often use the label in circumstances in which a person is behaving in unusual or dangerous ways. Such behaviours include

Caring for People with Learning Disabilities. Edited by I. Peate and D. Fearns.

self-injury, aggression, destruction of the environment, sexually inappropriate acts, fire-setting, faecal smearing and others. In such circumstances, challenging behaviour is very real.

DEFINING CHALLENGING BEHAVIOUR

Prior to discussing any issues pertaining to challenging behaviour, it is essential to refer to definitions of challenging behaviour, in order to establish a framework to help carers who assist adults with challenging behaviour, and to identify those who are labelled as having 'challenging' behaviours.

Challenging behaviour, by definition, presents carers with difficult emotional and professional challenges. The term 'challenging behaviour' has been defined as:

'. . . culturally abnormal behaviour(s) of such an intensity or duration that the physical safety of the person or others is likely to be placed in serious jeopardy, or behaviour which is likely to seriously limit use of or result in the person being denied access to ordinary community facilities.'

(Emerson et al. 1988)

The Department of Health (1993) pointed out that any successful interventions rely on staff/carers having a broad knowledge base in relation to safe reactive strategies, psychological and behavioural approaches and long-term skills-teaching strategies. Skills and knowledge linked with behaviour are central in managing challenging behaviour and have been shown to be effective (Lindsay 2001). It is useful to have an overview of a range of definitions; these are presented in Table 3.1.

Many carers refer to challenging behaviour as a specific behaviour or a group of behaviours which involve significant risks to people's physical well-being, or which act to reduce access to community settings, or result in being denied access to ordinary community facilities. These may include, for example, exhibiting physical and verbal aggression and perhaps minor self-injury and stereotyping behaviours which may lead to significant levels of avoidance by members of the public. It should be noted that challenging behaviour is not synonymous with mental health or psychiatric disorder, but appears to be a functional adaptive response to particular environments, people and objects, for example, rather than the manifestation of any underlying psychiatric pathological impairment. As Blunden and Allen (1987) point out, the term 'challenging behaviour':

'. . . emphasises that such behaviour represents challenges to services rather than problems with individuals with intellectual disabilities in some way carry around with them.'

(Blunden & Allen 1987, p. 14)

Table 3.1. An overview of a range of definitions concerning challenging behaviour

Author/researcher	Year	Definition
Emerson, E. et al.	1998	abnormal behaviour of such an intensity,
Emerson, E.	1996	frequency or duration that the physical safety of the person or others is likely to be placed in jeopardy . . .
Hastings, R. P. et al.	1997	challenging behaviour is an intentional behaviour with deliberate expectations . . .
Hastings R. P. et al.	1994	behaviour can be seen as deliberate and is likely to cause negative emotions and responses in staff
Carr, E. G. et al.	1991	attributions have also been said to influence staff confidence about their ability to manage challenging behaviour and argues that these beliefs can overshadow staff knowledge, leading to inappropriate responses to challenging behaviour
Blunden, R. & Allen, D.	1987	challenging behaviour/s emphasises that such behaviours represent challenges to the services rather than problems which individuals with intellectual disabilities in some way carry around them
Slee, R.	1996	in challenging behaviour the practice should be interpreted as how a person labelled as having challenging behaviour will be treated and where they will be treated
Gates, R.	2005	challenging behaviour is any behaviour that presents challenges because of its problematic and assumptive responses to the carers. The term challenging behaviour has come to define a disparate group of people and behaviours that seem to be ever increasing

Many people are unaware of the implications of definition and therefore the label challenging behaviour is often misused or misinterpreted. As Gates (1997) stated, it may well be that the term is used as a euphemism for, or an attempt to sanitise, what some regard as unacceptable behaviour, implying that the ownership of such behaviour therefore must reside with the individual displaying it.

In many senses, it is preferable to think about people's behaviours in terms of the thoughts and feelings which generate them. However, 'challenging behaviour' is the popular, universal term currently in use, and this is the one used throughout this chapter.

To construe a situation as a challenge rather than a problem encourages more constructive responses, although it would, of course, be mistaken to believe that minor changes in terminology are capable of bringing about major changes in practice.

The spectrum of challenging behaviour as adapted from Nihira et al. (1993) is a portrayal of negative behaviours which often are used as definitions, such as:

- violence
- rebelliousness
- destructiveness
- stereotypical behaviour
- unacceptable eccentric habits
- hyperactivity
- sexually non-socially accepted behaviour
- peculiar mannerisms and mimicries
- SIB (self-injurious behaviour)
- untrustworthiness
- emotional/psychological disturbances.

AETIOLOGY AND CAUSATION OF CHALLENGING BEHAVIOUR

In the previous section, definitions of challenging behaviours have been discussed. This section provides a brief outline of the causative factors that may contribute to the development of challenging behaviour. The cause of challenging behaviour is not a single factor but is often an amalgamation of several or all of the following factors:

- physical
- biological
- behavioural
- environmental
- psychological.

In many cases, it is the combination of one and more factors that gives rise to someone being stigmatised or labelled as having negative and difficult behaviour.

Challenging behaviour is both relatively common and relatively persistent amongst people with learning disabilities. British studies (Harris & Oliver 1992; Qureshi & Alborz 1992) have suggested that rates are not directly comparable (because of the different behaviours considered and definitions used) but they show the extent of the problem. Qureshi and Alborz's 1992 study suggests that in an area with a population of 220,000, we can expect between 31 and 56 people to present significant challenging behaviour.

Reeves (1997) has commented that learning disabled people may have identifiable neurological dysfunctions which are often misinterpreted as

Table 3.2. Some key points in relation to challenging behaviour

---

CHALLENGING BEHAVIOUR
- In general, challenging behaviour is seen as serving a necessary purpose for an individual.
- Challenging behaviours are largely learned behaviours. These are learned through interaction with others or the environment.
- Challenging behaviour may be a means through which the individual attempts to communicate any unmet needs.
- Any individual behaviour may be maintained by a variety of differing outcomes.
- A group of behaviours may be used to achieve a single outcome.

---

challenging behaviour and are therefore left untreated. The exploration of the physical causations of challenging behaviour indicates that some phenotypes and biological dysfunctions may result in behavioural difficulties and only account for a limited number of cases. If physical causes are identified, steps must be taken to alleviate the symptoms. Table 3.2 provides a brief outline of challenging behaviour.

SUMMARY OF CHALLENGING BEHAVIOUR

When dealing with challenging behaviour, it is important to recognise the range of behaviours which challenge services, and the effect that these behaviours have on both adults with learning disabilities and those who support them.

These behaviours have causes, many of which are identifiable and many of which are related to either the adult with learning disability's needs or the adult with a learning disability being unable to communicate his/her needs effectively.

Careful and comprehensive assessment of the causes and functions of behaviour is essential. Interactions which are designed to respond to the behaviour should be non-aversive (i.e. punishment of challenging behaviour is not the intervention of choice).

Ways of responding to challenging behaviour include:

- Careful analysis of the environment to ensure that it supports appropriate, rather than challenging behaviour.
- Helping adults with learning disabilities to learn new skills and more appropriate ways of expressing their needs.
- Trying 'treatment' of the behaviour, with advice from other professionals, such as strategies for strengthening appropriate behaviour and weakening inappropriate behaviour.

- Ensuring that staff know how to react in accordance with clear and agreed guidelines when the challenging behaviour does occur.

Challenging behaviour will probably not 'go away', although, with a reasoned response, it may reduce. Therefore, ways of working with adults with learning disabilities who exhibit challenging behaviour need to remain in place permanently.

Long-term, effective support for staff working with adults with learning disabilities who exhibit challenging behaviour is essential, as working in these situations is often stressful and difficult.

ASSESSING CHALLENGING BEHAVIOUR

Adults with learning disabilities who have challenging behaviour present acute management problems. Families and carers are often highly stressed and there is a huge temptation to use medication as an intervention. The aim of an intervention is to create and sustain the conditions under which the individual is most likely to be able to function. Challenging behaviour is functional; it may be an indication of physical discomfort, pain, emotional distress, mental illness or conflicts in the person's environment. A person's behaviour will be defined as challenging when it is judged by another to be socially unacceptable and when it evokes significant negative emotional responses in the other.

However, functional analysis will generate action plans which yield gains in personal well-being and behaviour functioning. Gates (2003) defines functional analysis as 'a process of seeking to understand the relationship between the various stimuli in the environment and the shaping and maintenance of behaviour through reinforcement'.

THE ASSESSMENT OF THE BEHAVIOUR

The starting point is a referral. Functional assessment is a range of strategies used to identify the antecedents and consequences that control challenging behaviour. Slevin (1999) defines it as a process for gathering information that can be used to maximise the effectiveness and efficiency of support. It focuses on the person and the environment in which the behaviour is occurring, takes into account the life of the person, helps to identify factors that contribute to the behaviour and helps to understand why the behaviour is occurring. There are approaches to functional assessment which comprise the following factors:

- Defining a specific behaviour of concern: individuals identified as challenging may do several things that cause concern. A productive outcome is more likely with one specific concern as the starting point.
- Assessing the immediate circumstances that surround specific incidents of the behaviour: antecedents – these are events that happened during the period before a behaviour that need to be modified. These are called triggers and/or stimuli and may increase the likelihood of the behaviour re-occurring. This may be done by:
  1. interviewing those involved with the person's care or the person himself;
  2. getting staff and carers to keep structured records of incidents, e.g. Antecendents, Behaviour, Consequences (ABC) charts or incident analysis forms (see Table 3.3);
  3. using an external observer to record incidents with scatterplot charts, such as the Motivation Assessment Scale (MAS).
- Assessing the individual: a detailed history will be required. Assessment of the key areas of individual functioning will involve detailed observations and a range of specialist assessments, such as Strategic Alternative Learning Techniques (SALT 2002/3). These will help to answer the question 'What is reinforcing the behaviour?' and identify the function of the behaviour to provide useful information to compile a functional strategy for working with the behaviour.

Table 3.3. ABC Incident Analysis (Source: LaVigna & Willis 1995)

Name:								
ABC Observation Sheet								
Date	Time Start	Time Finish	Those Present	Location	**ANTECEDENT** *What happened before*	**BEHAVIOUR** *Exactly what happened*	**CONSEQUENCE** *What happened afterwards*	Your name

- Assessing characteristics of individuals' living environments: usually by observation and discussion with the person and others with whom s/he lives and works. Data are collected to confirm whether events that predict behaviour are accurate and hypotheses about the function of the behaviour are correct.

SOME REASONS FOR CHALLENGING BEHAVIOUR

There may be several reasons why a person presents with challenging behaviour. Below is a list outlining some of these reasons:

- biological causes of challenging behaviour;
- challenging behaviour as a response to a poor environment;
- challenging behaviour as learnt behaviour;
- challenging behaviour as a communicative act;
- challenging behaviour as a response to emotional trauma;
- challenging behaviour as part of a mental illness.

FOUR RESPONSE CLASSES FOR CHALLENGING BEHAVIOUR

Attention
  People can engage in problem behaviour to get another person to attend to or spend time with them. Attention can be verbal, physical, social or related to proximity. The length of attention can vary.
Tangible
  A person wants to access an item, service, food/drink or activity. Gaining materials and activities that positive behaviour may not be so effective in accessing may positively reinforce challenging behaviour.
Sensory
  This provides input into one or more sensory-perceived pathways. Looks, sounds, smells, tastes or feels good or otherwise produces pleasure for the person. Challenging behaviour may be positively reinforced by the automatic sensory or perceptual consequence of the behaviour.
Escape
  The escape or avoidance of a request, task or activity can negatively reinforce problem behaviour. If problem behaviour occurs more often under these conditions, it is inferred that the behaviour occurs to escape the demand.

In Table 3.4, the factors that contribute to challenging behaviours are detailed.

Table 3.4. Factors which contribute to challenging behaviour

Adults with learning disabilities
- Mental health problems
- Personal stress
- Recent crisis
- Expecting interaction to be difficult because of previous experience
- Young people possibly less control because of immaturity
- Presence of a particular individual
- Positive feedback from peers
- Tiredness

Carer factors
- Health, overwork, stress and reduced tolerance
- Age
- Experience
- Sex
- Personality
- Temperament
- Attitudes
- Workload
- Shift work
- Appearance

Interaction factors
- Giving bad news
- Correcting behaviour
- Providing personal care
- Withdrawal of service
- Inflexible routines

Situational factors
- Temperature of environment
- Working alone
- Transporting someone in your car alone
- Time of day
- Noise level
- Increased number of people
- Moving between settings
- Task/activity too difficult for individual

Case study
Concepts of challenging behaviour
   John is sitting quite happily in the sitting room. He likes spending time alone. Someone comes along and asks him to go into the dining room and guides him there. As soon as the request to move is made, John begins to slap himself and starts screaming. He bites his right fist and hits the wall.

What is the cause/trigger? Perhaps he:

- does not like the person
- does not like the dining room
- was interested in what was on TV
- does not like the food he knows he is going to get
- has a pain in his stomach and does not want to eat
- does not like the person he will have to sit beside at the table
- feels anxious about a training programme designed to help him feed himself.

ACTION: Identify and discuss possible triggers and behaviours resulting from these triggers.

SOME TIPS FOR CARING FOR ADULTS WITH LEARNING DISABILITIES AND CHALLENGING BEHAVIOUR

Challenging behaviour is any behaviour that interferes with the adult with a learning disability's learning development and success in daily routines or activities; is harmful to the adult with a learning disability and other people; or puts the adult with a learning disability at high risk for later problems and failures.

Caring for an adult with a learning disability with challenging behaviour is a challenge in its own right – but it is one that carers can overcome with the appropriate strategies. Table 3.5 offers some ideas that have been proven to work and which can benefit all adults with learning disabilities, not just those with challenging behaviour.

Some key points related to John and his behaviour are as follows. When someone like John is unmanageable or out of control, it appears that nothing is working out:

- Stand between John and the rest of the world – keep a safe distance and do not become physical by trying to move or handle him.
- Do not confront him. To keep him from feeling trapped, stand aside, remain composed and do not stare into his eyes.
- Do not talk or shout, as John is not ready to listen.
- Do not ignore his behaviour, but when he is calm, talk to him quietly. Assist him in expressing his feelings. Try to show him that people care for him and assist him in coping with problem strategies for next time.
- Establish an ABC (Antecedent, Behaviour, Consequence) Behaviour Chart (Felce & McBrien 1992).

Table 3.5. Some ideas that may enhance care for all people with learning disabilities, not only those with challenging behaviour

Caring for the adult with a learning disability – be sure that she or he knows that you care for him/her and set aside time to spend with him/her.

Give him/her your undivided attention and let him/her have a choice; let him/her choose his/her own activity and make sure she or he knows you appreciate his/her input in activities.

Appropriate behaviour – this must be encouraged, thus minimising the opportunities for challenging behaviours. It is important to build appropriate patterns of behaviour so that trouble can be anticipated, to prevent the difficult situation from occurring and help the adult with a learning disability to remember what to do instead of correcting his/her mistakes.

The environment provided must enhance success and opportunities. Safety must be of primary importance, i.e. remove any dangerous objects, fragile items. Try to provide comfortable areas of activities and select items that interest the adult with a learning disability with challenging behaviour. Use inclusion techniques and keep all activities well planned and organised.

Pick activities around the needs of the individual, e.g. if Mary is very upset when she is painting because she is hungry, give her a snack.

Set goals and clear limits, and enforce them consistently. Attempt to encourage the adult with a learning disability with challenging behaviour to know what is expected. Certain allowances should be made, such as Mary leaving her paintbrush on the table – that's OK.

Create opportunities/routines and stick to them. Adults with learning disabilities and challenging behaviour like routines and predictability, especially when they know what's coming next. It is also important to give some advance instructions of changes in activity, e.g. 'After you go for a walk, you must have your tea'.

As a carer, learn to recognise changes in mood, especially with anxiety levels. As a carer, stop the task you are doing and give more attention to the adult with a learning disability whom you are caring for, e.g. give him a smile or ask if you can help or listen to him carefully. If you can prevent a problem in good time and in the early stages, then challenging behaviour may be prevented.

Do not discourage activities by saying 'Don't do it', but ask whether he wishes to do something else. Be patient if he needs this support repeatedly, and allow him to practise.

From an empathy point of view, as a carer, put yourself in someone's shoes and try to find out how he gets what he wants from his challenging behaviour. Does he get attention (positive or negative)? Does he do it to avoid things? Is he calmer? Once you identify the challenging behaviour, then you can help the adult with a learning disability to cope in a more acceptable way.

Remain calm. When things are not going smoothly, take a deep breath and count to 10. By showing the adult with a learning disability that you can handle the situation with a cool and tolerant head, you can become his role model.

UNDERSTANDING CHALLENGING BEHAVIOUR

Frameworks for understanding challenging behaviour have become more sophisticated over time, with important implications for assessment and intervention practices. These frameworks will be illustrated and their implications considered. An example of the assessment and intervention planning process will be illustrated. It is well recognised that 'demands' often set off challenging behaviour. If an adult with a learning disability is asked to wash the floor, s/he may become aggressive. This often results in action to calm the person down or prevent injury to him/herself or others. The adult with a learning disability may be moved to another room or restrained, or prescribed medication and so on. In any event, s/he ends up not washing the floor. One of the earliest sensible conceptions of challenging behaviour depicted exactly this pattern (see Figure 3.1).

The demand 'sets off' aggression, which results in escape from the demand. From the perspective of the carer (Figure 3.2), the person's aggression 'sets off' their removing the demand and the aggression stops (with some luck)!

The outcome of this process can be readily seen. The adult with a learning disability is more likely to become aggressive when presented with demands and the carer is more likely to remove demands when s/he becomes aggressive.

Whatever the exact nature of the 'thought', s/he is likely to be feeling distressed and wanting to get rid of his/her distress. Aggressive behaviour may then succeed in removing both the demand and (eventually) his/her own distress, as shown in Figure 3.3.

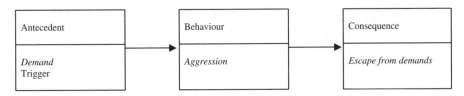

Figure 3.1. The ABC model of challenging behaviour

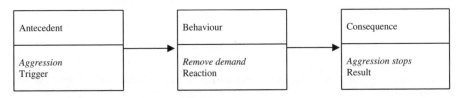

Figure 3.2. Challenging behaviour from the perspective of the carer

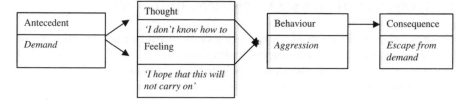

Figure 3.3. A model of challenging behaviour which takes into account thoughts and feelings

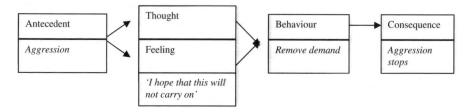

Figure 3.4. A model of challenging behaviour which takes into account the carer's thoughts and feelings

The carer may well have similar thoughts and feelings, s/he may be thinking (negatively) that sh/e does not know how to cope with the person's behaviour and s/he is almost certainly feeling distressed and frightened (see Figure 3.4).

This extension of these models helps us to feel that we can understand the motivation of the two parties better, and shows how negative thoughts and feelings may have maladaptive consequences. Given this depiction, it would not be surprising to find that both parties developed failure sets about these kinds of interactions (and therefore avoided them if at all possible), and both parties learned to handle their distress by seeking to escape from the distressing situation.

Expanded models may develop from the above, bearing in mind that four kinds of background factors are included: temporary personal (such as feeling tired), persistent personal (such as difficulty in understanding speech), temporary environmental (such as a lot of noise) and persistent environmental (such as a climate of social control).

The aim of any intervention is to interrupt the sequence leading to the adults with learning disabilities exhibiting challenging behaviour as early as possible, so that difficulties are prevented, not just reacted to, and to develop skills to cope better with the difficulties being faced. The intervention includes:

1. Making realistic demands based on information of skill.
2. Anticipating difficulties.
3. Developing skills (coping strategies for dealing with problems, training in recognising and dealing with distress).
4. Support for carers (guidance for preventing and managing difficulties and also joint approaches).

CONCLUDING COMMENTS ON CHALLENGING BEHAVIOUR

When dealing with challenging behaviour, it is important to recognise the range of behaviours which challenge services, and the effect that these behaviours have on both adults with learning disabilities and those who support them.

Bear in mind that behaviours have causes, many of which are identifiable and many of which are related to either the needs of adults with learning disabilities or their inability to communicate these needs effectively. Careful and comprehensive assessment of the causes and functions of behaviour is essential, as are interactions which are designed to respond to the behaviour, which should be non-aversive (i.e. punishment of challenging behaviour is not the intervention of choice).

There are many ways of responding to challenging behaviour and they include:

- Careful analysis of the environment to ensure that it supports appropriate, rather than challenging, behaviour.
- Helping adults with learning disabilities to learn new skills and more appropriate ways of expressing their needs.
- Trying 'treatment' of the behaviour, with advice from other professionals, e.g. strategies for strengthening appropriate behaviour and weakening inappropriate behaviour.
- Ensuring that carers know how to react in accordance with clear and agreed guidelines when the challenging behaviour does occur.

Challenging behaviour will probably not 'go away', although, with a reasoned response, it may reduce. Therefore, ways of working with adults with learning disabilities with challenging behaviour need to remain in place permanently.

Long-term, effective support for carers working with adults with learning disabilities with challenging behaviour is essential, as working with these situations is often stressful and difficult.

Overall:

- We need people with the skills to conduct this process. As the number of people with such skills is currently rather limited, significant investment in training is required; this must be consistent and pragmatic.
- We need to develop (or identify) model services which can support training and allow more extensive evaluation and development of the approach.
- We need services which are receptive to the approach. This involves both shared understanding about the nature of challenging behaviour and a willingness to make the sorts of changes to service practices which are required.
- We need appropriate research programmes and data gathering for reflective and evaluative analysis.

Finally, it is hoped that in combining the above and outlining some understanding of challenging behaviours, we will create a potential to improve progressively the lifestyles of adults with learning disabilities at risk of challenging behaviour and support their full inclusion, creating valued lives in the community with appropriate social standards.

ACKNOWLEDGEMENT

A big thank you to my wife Laura and son Nikos – two very special people in my life – and my father for all my inspiration and career guidance and my mother for being Mum. Also to my colleagues from the University of Hertfordshire for giving me this opportunity to contribute to this book.

REFERENCES

Blunden, R. & Allen, D. (1987) *Facing the Challenge: An Ordinary Life for People with Learning Disabilities and Challenging Behaviour*, King's Fund paper no. 74, Kings Fund Centre, London.

Carr, E. G. et al. (1991) 'The Effects of Severe Behaviour Problems in Children on the Teaching Behaviour in Adults', *Journal of Applied Behaviour Analysis*, **24**: 523–35.

Department of Health (1993) *Services for People with Learning Disabilities and Challenging Behaviours or Mental Health Needs*, Report of the Protech Group, London, HMSO.

Emerson, E. (1996) 'Some Challenges Presented by Severe Self-Injurious Behaviour (SIB)', *Mental Handicap*, **17**: 92–8.

Emerson, E., Cummings, R., Barrett, S., Hughes, H., McCool, C. & Toogood, A. (1988) 'Challenging Behaviour and Community Services: Who are the People who Challenge Services?, *Mental Handicap*, **16**: 16–19.

Felce, D. & McBrien, J. (1992) *Working with People Who Have Severe Learning Difficulty and Challenging Behaviour*, Kidderminster, BIMH, NFER–Nelson Publishing.

Gates, B. (1997) 'Behavioural Difficulties', in B. Gates (ed.), *Learning Disabilities* Glasgow, Churchill Livingstone.

Gates, B. (2003) *Learning Disabilities: Towards Inclusion*, London, Churchill Livingstone, pp. 176 and 446.

Harris, P. & Oliver, R. (1992) 'How to Meet the Challenge', *Health Service Journal*, **8 October**: 28–9.

Hastings, R. P., Remmington, B. & Hopper, G. M. (1994) 'Experienced and Inexperienced Health Care Workers' Beliefs about Challenging Behaviours', *Journal of Intellectual Disability Research*, **39**(6): 22–34.

Hastings, R. P. et al. (1997) 'Community Staff Counsel Attributions about Challenging Behaviour in People with Intellectual Disabilities', *Journal of Applied Research in Intellectual Disabilities*, **10**(3): 238–49.

LaVigna, G. W. & Willis, T. J. (1995) 'Challenging Behaviour: A Model for Breaking the Barriers to Social and Community Integration', *Positive Practices*, **1**(1): 8–15.

Lindsay, W. R. (2001) 'Behavioural Disturbance', in L. Hamilton-Kirkwood (ed.), *Health Evidence Bulletins Wales: Learning Disabilities (Intellectual Disability)*, Cardiff, Cardiff National Assembly for Wales.

Nihira, K., Leland, H. & Lambert, N. (1993) *AAMR – Adaptive Behavior Scale Residential and Community Examiners' Manual*, 2nd edn, Pro. Texas.

Qureshi, H. & A. Alborz (1992) 'Epidemiology of Challenging Behaviour', in E. Emerson, P. McGill & J. Mansell (eds), *Severe Learning Disabilities and Challenging Behaviour: Designing High Quality Services*, London, Chapman and Hall.

Reeves, S. (1997) 'Behavioural Misdiagnosis', *Nursing Times*, **93**(19): 44–5.

SALT (2002/3) The Strategic Alternative Learning Techniques Center, The University of Arizona, SALT Center, PO Box 210136, Tuscon.

Slee, R. (1996) 'Clauses of Conditionality: The Reasonable Accommodation of Language', in L. Barton (ed.), *Disability and Society: Emerging Issues and Insights*, London, Longman.

Slevin, E. (1999) 'Challenging Behaviour', *Mental Health Care*, **1**(21).

USEFUL ADDRESSES

The information below includes internet websites and addresses of providers of information and training, which may be of interest to people wishing to explore issues relating to challenging behaviour.

The British Institute of Learning Disabilities (BILD),
Wolverhampton Road,
Kidderminster,
Worcestershire,
DY10 3PP,
UK.
Tel: 01562 850251; fax: 01562 851970

BILD provides a range of well-regarded and educational opportunities.

The Tizard Centre,
Beverley Farm,
University of Kent at Canterbury,
Canterbury,
Kent,
CT2 7LZ,
UK.
Tel: 01227 764000; fax: 01227 763674

The Tizard Centre has developed useful training packs for those wishing to educate others about how to understand challenging behaviour.

Pavilion Publishing and Conference Services,
Pavilion Publishing,
8 St George's Place,
Brighton,
Sussex,
BN1 4GB,
UK.
Tel: 01273 623222; fax: 01273 625526; http://www.pavpub.com

Pavilion Publishing provide useful information and training packs relating to challenging behaviour.

The East Yorkshire Learning Disability Institute (EYLDI),
The University of Hull,
Hull,
HU6 7RX,
UK.
Tel: 01482 465241; fax: 01482 466699; www.hull.ac.uk/Hull/health.ps/ld/eyld.
htm

EYLDI offers consultancy and training on the subject of challenging behaviour.

4 Protecting 'Vulnerable' Adults with Learning Disabilities

DEBRA FEARNS

KEY POINTS

- The abuse of vulnerable adults with learning disabilities is a difficult and disturbing area; the carer requires a high degree of sensitivity, skill and knowledge to address the issue effectively.
- Good quality service provision will ensure that people with additional and complex needs are appropriately cared for.
- Those vulnerable adults with learning disabilities often have other associated health problems.
- All adults should be able to live free from fear and harm, as well as having their rights and choices protected, and this includes those adults with learning disabilities.

INTRODUCTION

Since the late 1950s and 1960s, there has been a growing shift and change in the way in which Western society views adults with learning disabilities and those with mental health needs. Goffman's (1961) seminal work, *Asylums*, highlighted the bleak, unfulfilling lives of many adults with mental health needs, exposing the inhuman and degrading conditions that were present in many long-stay hospitals that catered for mentally ill people or those with learning disabilities. Goffman (1961) used the term 'institutionalisation' to convey the ways in which adults became depersonalised by the systems designed to care for them, including the staff who were meant to provide care in their everyday lives. Goffman (1961) identified a set of features that defined aspects of institutionalisation, including depersonalisation, block treatment, rigid, inflexible systems of care and social detachment between the staff and those he termed as 'inmates'.

Adults with learning disabilities have a long history of exclusion, segregation and abuse. Often, this abuse was either ignored or denied, and carers

Caring for People with Learning Disabilities. Edited by I. Peate and D. Fearns.
Copyright © 2006 by John Wiley & Sons, Ltd.

were reluctant to acknowledge that it was happening. It is only during the past 40 years that attempts to change the lives of adults with learning disabilities for the better have had an impact. Segregation allowed these abuses to remain a hidden secret within long-stay hospitals – the primary home of vulnerable adults with learning disabilities. These concerns were boldly stated in *The Report of the Committee of Inquiry into Ely Hospital* (Howe Report 1969). This report highlighted the rundown provision, poor quality of care and degrading treatment that were present in the worst institutions. In 1975, a committee was set up by the government to investigate these conditions, resulting in the Jay Report (Jay Committee 1979). It recommended both local authority care, thus suggesting a move away from health provision, and developing services based on the values of 'normalisation'.

Wolfensberger's (1972) *Principle of Normalisation* outlined that services should be designed by those people using them. 'Normalisation' was taken to mean providing services that 'ordinary' people had access to, such as schooling and housing. However, it was to be nearly 20 years before it became accepted government policy to close down long-stay institutions that cared for those with learning disabilities and mental health needs in England and Wales. The White Paper *Caring for People* (Department of Health 1989) outlined the Government's obligation to close long-stay hospitals and instead develop health and social care services at a local level. The NHS and Community Care Act 1990 helped to provide assistance for people to live in their own homes, if at all possible. This was more commonly referred to as 'community care', and led to the permanent closure of many such institutions. Adults with learning disabilities, and also those with mental health needs, were 'resettled' into local communities, often at the expense of long-cherished friendships formed over many years. The belief was that living in small group homes, within local communities, would provide a better quality of life and might lead to greater acceptance within society, as they would no longer be segregated. This translated into services being developed locally to support individual choice, as advocated by O'Brien and Tyne (1989), based on the 5 Accomplishments for Service Provision. For many adults with learning disabilities, these have been positive changes, but we need to be alert to the possibility of 'mini-institutions' developing in some services that may hinder individual choice, freedom and inclusion.

CURRENT POSITION OF ADULTS WITH LEARNING DISABILITIES

The reality for many adults with learning disabilities is a life with limited choice, rights, independence or inclusion – the four key principles at the heart of *Valuing People* (Department of Health 2001b). This state of affairs puts many adults with learning disabilities in a vulnerable position, as they are dependent on family, carers and professionals to help them live their lives. This can lead to potential vulnerability, as an adult with a learning disability is reliant on the honesty, integrity and professionalism of those caring for him/her. Alongside this is the difficulty that adults with learning disabilities may have in making their needs and wishes known, and in being heard, listened to and understood by families, carers and professionals (Department of Health 2001b):

> 'People with learning disabilities are amongst the most socially excluded and vulnerable groups in Britain today. Very few have jobs, live in their own homes or have real choice over who cares for them. Many have few friends outside their families and those paid to care for them. Their voices are rarely heard in public. This needs to change.'
>
> (Department of Health 2001b, p. 14)

Whilst there may have been key changes made in the delivery and provision of some services that support adults with learning disabilities, the reality is that this has had little impact on overcoming obstacles that relate to social exclusion and access to services, facilities, housing and employment. This continued exclusion adds to the vulnerable position that many adults with learning disabilities find themselves in.

Emerson and Malam (2005) carried out a national survey of adults with learning disabilities and their families, in England. This survey highlights that adults with learning disabilities are often socially excluded. 43 per cent stated that they had been bullied at school; 32 per cent stated that they did not feel safe in either their homes, their locality, or whilst using public transport; and 32 per cent also stated that someone had been rude or offensive to them in the last year, because they had a learning disability. Worryingly, 9 per cent stated that they had been the victim of crime in the preceding year.

Activity 1:
What barriers can you identify that you think may cause an adult with a learning disability to feel socially excluded?
What steps could you take to reduce social exclusion and vulnerability?

DEFINITION OF 'VULNERABLE ADULTS'

What do we mean when we talk about 'vulnerable adults'? *The New Oxford English Dictionary* defines it as: 'exposed to the possibility of being attacked or harmed, either physically or emotionally'.

The Department of Health's guidance (Department of Health 2000) defined it thus:

'The broad definition of a "vulnerable adult" referred to in the 1997 Consultation Paper *Who Decides?*, issued by the Lord Chancellor's Department, is a person:

'who is or may be in need of community care services by reason of mental or other disability, age or illness; and who is or may be unable to take care of him or herself, or unable to protect him or herself against significant harm or exploitation.'

(Department of Health 2000, Section 2.3)

PROTECTION OF VULNERABLE ADULTS WITH LEARNING DISABILITIES

In recent years, there has been growing recognition that adults with learning disabilities, and those who have a mental illness or who are old and frail, need protection from potentially abusive situations over which they may have little control. In light of this, following on from the consultation publication of *No Secrets* (Department of Health 2000), the 'Protection of Vulnerable Adults Scheme in England and Wales for Care Homes and Domiciliary Care Agencies' was implemented by the Department of Health in 2004. It outlines best practice guidance that needs to be put in place to protect vulnerable adults. This guidance also includes changes that have been made to the need for Criminal Records Bureau Disclosures. This Protection of Vulnerable Adults scheme is more commonly known as POVA. The central tenet is to protect vulnerable adults by ensuring that potential care staff are screened to prevent those who have a poor track record of care or those who may intend to harm vulnerable adults from gaining employment. The POVA scheme is set out in the Care Standards Act 2000, and at its centre is the POVA List. The POVA List will enable care staff to be both checked against this list and have referrals made to this list. Therefore, care workers who have had previous incidents of harming a vulnerable adult or have placed a vulnerable adult at risk of harm (whether this is while they are employed or not) will be banned from being employed to care for a vulnerable adult. The term 'employment' is used to describe paid, unpaid and voluntary work.

Under section 121 of the Care Standards Act 2000, the term 'harm' is defined as:

'. . . in relation to an adult who is not mentally impaired, means ill treatment or the impairment of health; and
in relation to an adult who is mentally impaired, or a child, means ill treatment or the impairment of health or development.'

The POVA scheme does not apply to the National Health Service (NHS) and independent healthcare sector, but they will be brought on line as soon as is practical, as set out in the Care Standards Act 2000.

The definition of a 'vulnerable adult' in section 80(6) of the Care Standards Act 2000 states that:

'Vulnerable adult' means:

a. 'an adult to whom accommodation and nursing or personal care are provided in a care home;
b. an adult to whom personal care is provided in their own home under arrangements made by a domiciliary care agency.'

There is now greater legislative protection afforded to vulnerable adults, as it has been evident over a number of years that specific legislation and guidance had been lacking in protecting vulnerable adults with learning disabilities from abuse and crime.

No Secrets (Department of Health 2000) offers useful definitions of six categories of abuse and how they might impact on individuals:

- '**Physical abuse**, including hitting, slapping, pushing, kicking, misuse of medication, restraint, or inappropriate sanctions;
- **Sexual abuse**, including rape and sexual assault or sexual acts to which the vulnerable adult has not consented, or could not consent or was pressured into consenting;
- **Psychological abuse**, including emotional abuse, threats of harm or abandonment, deprivation of contact, humiliation, blaming, controlling, intimidation, coercion, harassment, verbal abuse, isolation or withdrawal from services or supportive networks;
- **Financial or material abuse**, including theft, fraud, exploitation, pressure in connection with wills, property or inheritance or financial transactions, or the misuse or misappropriation of property, possessions or benefits;
- **Neglect and acts of omission**, including ignoring medical or physical care needs, failure to provide access to appropriate health, social care or educational services, the withholding of the necessities of life, such as medication, adequate nutrition and heating; and
- **Discriminatory abuse**, including racist, sexist, that based on a person's disability, and other forms of harassment, slurs or similar treatment.'

(Department of Health 2000, p. 9)

No Secrets (Department of Health 2000) provides a very useful framework for supporting professionals to work in partnership with adults with learning disabilities, offering greater protection and security to those who most need it. It sets out that codes of practice should be developed by partnership working, with local authority social services departments taking the lead roles. This is because social services will be legally responsible for implementing the policy and procedures. Each local authority will devise its own policies and procedures, in consultation with other relevant agencies, such as the police, health and housing. The implementation of the framework policy and procedures will be monitored by the Commission for Social Care Inspectorate (CSCI).

THE LEGAL FRAMEWORK FOR PROTECTING VULNERABLE ADULTS

The regulations relating to the ill-treatment of vulnerable adults with learning disabilities are often complex and not always easy to understand. However, laws are in place which can be used either to protect vulnerable adults or to act on their behalf if a crime or offence has been committed against them. It does require carers, students and professionals to have some knowledge of the law and knowledge of whom to contact for further assistance. If a criminal offence is suspected, it should always be referred to the police. Advice should always be sought from senior colleagues and managers on the next stages that should follow. 'Doing nothing' is not an option.

The sections outlined below are based on the definitions outlined in the *No Secrets* guidance (Department of Health 2000). The following list is not complete, but is meant to denote laws that can help and support vulnerable adults with learning disabilities, and offer them protection within a legal framework.

PHYSICAL ABUSE

Assault

An offence of common assault is committed when a person assaults another person. Assault also takes account of both behaviour and language, so that any acts or words in connection with the use or threat of immediate violence to another person may signify assault.

Battery

An offence of battery is committed when a person intentionally and recklessly applies unlawful force to another. It carries a maximum penalty of six months' imprisonment and/or a fine not exceeding the statutory maximum.

Assault occasioning actual bodily harm: section 47 of the Offences Against the Person Act 1861

This is defined by the degree of injury and the sentences available to the court. A key factor here would be:

'b. the vulnerability of the victim, such as when the victim is elderly, disabled or a child assaulted by an adult ... the charge will normally be assault occasioning actual bodily harm.'

(Assault Occasioning Grievous Bodily Harm, sections 18 and 20,
Offences Against the Person Act 1861)

Affray: section 3(1) of the Public Order Act 1986

This offence involves the use of threatening violence to another person and the other person fearing for his/her personal safety.

Fear or provocation of violence: section 4(1) of the Public Order Act 1986

This may involve threatening, abusive or insulting words and behaviour to another person, or threatening, abusive or insulting signs, writing or other visible representations that provoke unlawful violence or where the other person fears that unlawful violence will be used against them.

Restraint or the threat of restraint can amount to an assault or battery. It can also include any practice involving physical force, such as force-feeding. In addition, the human rights of the person may also be infringed, under the Human Rights Act 1998.

The detention of an adult against his/her wishes can constitute false imprisonment. In addition, specific guidance exists to protect adults with learning disabilities from physical restraint, as outlined by Harris et al. (1996). In addition, further advice suggests that:

'Professionals working with vulnerable people have a duty of care to ensure that in this context it means a need to avoid actions that may harm others, and that the agencies they work for act always in the best interest of the service user. Also, the framework provided by criminal and civil law should ensure that people can live without "interference from others" including for example assault or false imprisonment.'

(Powell & Northfield 2002)

These laws can offer a measure of protection for adults with learning disabilities if the incidents are reported as crimes and prosecuted effectively. Identifying and supporting adults with learning disabilities who are vulnerable as victims or perpetrators of crime by police officers are also problematic, with many police officers' relying on intuition and appearance, amongst other unreliable factors (Fearns 2001). When combined with some professionals working within the criminal justice system's having a limited understanding of the needs of disabled adults, it is not difficult to understand why some believe that they will not be 'credible' witnesses. As Clare and Murphy (2001) point out, too:

'. . . people with learning disabilities themselves need to be empowered to recognise, and respond to crime and other types of anti-social behaviour against themselves or others'.

SEXUAL ABUSE

Sexual Offences Act 2003

The Sexual Offences Act 2003 came into force on 1 May 2004, following extensive consultation and developing from the White Paper, *Protecting the Public* (Department of Health 2002). The main purpose of the act is to modernise and strengthen the law relating to sexual offences; add enhanced preventative measures; and protect individuals from sexual offenders. It also contains a new definition of 'consent':

> '. . . a person consents if she/he agrees, by choice and has the freedom and capacity to make that choice.'
>
> (Sexual Offences Act 2003, section 74)

The Sexual Offences Act places the emphasis on victims first. It contains new offences in which the victim is considered to have a mental disorder, and it targets a wider range of exploitative behaviours. These include: sexual touching including penetration, causing/inciting a person to engage in sexual activity, engaging in sexual activity in their presence, causing a person to watch the action. The act uses the current definition of 'mental disorder' from the Mental Health Act 1983, which is:

> 'Mental disorder means mental illness, arrested or incomplete development of mind, psychopathic disorder and any other disorder or disability of mind and "mentally disordered" shall be construed accordingly.'

A person with a learning disability falls within the definition of mental disorder.

To prove that a person has a mental disorder, medical evidence will usually be required.

Offences involving sexual activity when mental disorder impedes choice are covered in sections 30–33, and primarily relate to profoundly disabled people. The defendant has to have knowledge of the victim's mental disorder, prior to conviction. This can either be specific knowledge or reasonable knowledge. If the victim is unable to refuse because of insufficient understanding or is unable to communicate, the defendant will receive a tough sentence.

Sections 34–37 relate to mental disorder, where inducement, threats or deception are used to procure sexual activity. In this instance, the issue of consent is irrelevant, but the defendant must have knowledge of the person's mental disorder.

Sections 38–41 relate to sexual activity between a person with a mental disorder and a care worker. A relationship of care, involving regular face-to-face contact, needs to be established, whether the person is employed or not. It is presumed that the defendant knows that the victim has a mental disorder. The prime function of these offences relates to the prosecution of those who have the capacity to consent, but, due to their mental disorder, may allow sexual activity only because they are predisposed to do so by their intimacy with and/or dependency on the carer. A defence can be mounted where there is a pre-existing sexual relationship, or where lawfully married (Pringle 2006).

The Sexual Offences Act 2003 means that there is stronger management of convicted sex offenders in the community. There is the Sexual Offences Prevention Order and the Risk of Harm Order. Both are civil orders, but if they are breached, they become criminal offences.

PSYCHOLOGICAL ABUSE

Harassment: section 1 of the Protection from Harassment Act 1997

This states that one individual must not pursue a course of conduct which amounts to harassment of another individual and which the person knows, or should know, amounts to harassment of the other person.

To bring a criminal prosecution, a 'course of conduct' must involve such behaviour on at least two occasions. Such behaviour can include verbal abuse. Civil action can also be taken by obtaining an injunction against the harasser (section 3). This is irrespective of whether a prosecution is brought against the harasser, or if previous harassment has taken place.

Under section 4 of the same act, a course of behaviour that on at least two occasions causes another person to fear that violence will be used against him/her can be an offence. In this case, the court has the power to issue a restraining order or injunction against the offender.

Under section 4A of the Public Order Act 1986, an offence is committed when a person intends to cause another harassment, alarm or distress by:

- 'using threatening, abusive or insulting words or behaviour, or disorderly behaviour, or
- displays any writing, sign or other visible representation which is threatening, abusive or insulting, thereby causing that or another person harassment, alarm or distress.

Section 5 covers similar offences without intent.

The Crime and Disorder Act 1998 allows for Anti-Social Behaviour Orders (ASBOs) to be applied for directly, by either the police or the local authority in consultation with each other. These may be particularly effective where adults with learning disabilities are being victimised by neighbours in their local community and, if these are breached, further action can be taken.

FINANCIAL/MATERIAL ABUSE

Theft is the dishonest appropriation of property belonging to another, with the intention of permanently depriving the owner of it (Theft Act 1968, section 2). Theft and dishonesty have to be proven. Under section 8 of the same act, robbery is theft aggravated by the use or threat of force.

Deception

There are a number of offences involving deception under the Theft Act 1968. These include obtaining property by deception and obtaining a pecuniary advantage by deception.

If a vulnerable adult with a learning disability is persuaded to enter into a contract that is clearly detrimental, such deception will usually annul the contract. The other party that persuaded the vulnerable adult could be charged with obtaining property by deception or obtaining a pecuniary advantage by deception.

Blackmail: section 21 of the Theft Act 1968

'A person is guilty of blackmail if, with a view to gain for himself or another or with intent to cause loss to another, he makes any unwarranted demand with menace; and for this purpose a demand with menaces is unwarranted unless the person making it does so in the belief:

(a) that he has reasonable grounds for making the demand; and
(b) that the use of menace is a proper means of reinforcing the demand.'

NEGLECT/OMISSION

The Mental Capacity Act 2005 became law on 7 April 2005, but will not be implemented until April 2007. The preamble to the act describes it as:

'An Act to make new provision relating to persons who lack capacity; to establish a superior court of record called the Court of Protection in place of the office of the Supreme Court called by that name; to make provision in connection with the Convention on the International Protection of Adults signed at the Hague on 13th January 2000; and for connected purposes.'

It provides a statutory framework to empower and protect vulnerable adults who may not be in a position to make their own decisions. Guidance on the act will be provided in a Statutory Code of Practice.

The Mental Capacity Act 2005 is underpinned by five key principles. These are:

- a presumption of capacity;
- the right for individuals to be supported to make their own decisions;
- the right for individuals to make what might be seen as eccentric or unwise decisions;
- best interests;
- least restrictive intervention of their basic rights and freedoms.

'The Act enshrines in statute current best practice and common law principles concerning people who lack mental capacity and those who take decisions on their behalf. It reforms and updates current statutory schemes for enduring powers of attorney and Court of Protection receivers.'

(Mental Capacity Act 2005)

The Mental Capacity Act 2005 also introduces a new criminal offence of ill-treatment or neglect of a person who lacks capacity. If found guilty, a defendant could expect a prison term of up to five years.

The issue of restraint is also covered in this act. It will be necessary to demonstrate that restraint is required to prevent harm, and that such restraint must be proportionate in terms of degree and duration of restraint. The onus is on the person carrying out the act of restraint to justify his/her belief that the person being restrained will suffer harm unless restrained. This can strengthen the protection afforded to adults with learning disabilities from physical restraint; this principle follows the spirit of Article 8 of the European Convention on Human Rights.

The National Assistance Act 1948, amended by the National Assistance Act 1951, under section 47, allows for the removal of people in need of care and attention. The criteria that need to be met are as follows, the:

- person is suffering from grave chronic disease or being aged and infirm or physically incapacitated, is living in insanitary conditions, and
- is unable to devote to themselves, and is not receiving proper care and attention
- removal from home is necessary, either in own interests, or preventing injury to health of, or serious nuisance to, other persons.

(National Assistance Act 1948, amended by
the National Assistance Act 1951)

The community physician, through the district council, applies, in writing, to the Magistrates' Court to remove the person from his/her home to ensure that s/he receives the care and attention that s/he requires. Although not used often, in can be used in cases in which there is serious neglect or self-neglect, but, under the Human Rights Act 1998, the power to detain a person for up to three weeks, without prior notice, may be deemed as infringing the person's human rights.

Section 287 of the Public Health Act 1936 does give local authorities the means to gain a warrant to enter and clean premises which represent a public health risk. This can be used to protect vulnerable adults who are unable to care for themselves or their accommodation to a 'reasonable' standard.

The Mental Health Act 1983 allows certain entry and inspection rights where it is believed that a person suffering from a mental disorder is living, if it is believed that s/he is not being cared for appropriately.

Under section 115 of the Mental Health Act 1983, an Approved Social Worker (ASW) may enter and inspect any accommodation where a person with a mental disorder is living, if s/he reasonably believes that the person is not under proper care. An ASW undergoes specific, specialist training in mental health issues and applying the Mental Health Act 1983, as well as initial qualification as a social worker. However, a warrant still needs to be obtained for forcible entry.

Section 135 of the Mental Health Act 1983 allows an application to be made to the Magistrates' Court for a warrant to search for and remove patients. This allows the police to enter the specified premises forcibly, if required to do so, to remove the person with a mental disorder to a place of safety.

The grounds for this are that there is reasonable cause to suspect that the person with a mental disorder:

- has been, or is being ill-treated, neglected or kept otherwise than under proper control, in any place within the court's jurisdiction; or
- being unable to care for him/herself is living alone in any such place.

This will enable further applications under the Mental Health Act 1983 to be made for his/her treatment or care. The place of safety may be a hospital, residential or nursing home, police station or another suitable place able to care for the patient.

Section 136 of this act – 'Mentally Disordered Persons Found in Public Places' – covers people found in public places. If a police officer finds a person in a public place who appears to be suffering from a mental disorder and to be in immediate need of care and control, the police officer may remove that person to a place of safety. This person may then be detained for up to 72 hours for the purpose of enabling him/her to be examined by a doctor and interviewed by an ASW. This also enables provision to be made, if necessary, for his/her treatment or care.

Section 7 of the Mental Health Act 1983 refers to guardianship. The guardian of a mentally disordered person has the power to require access to be given to the person under their guardianship, at any place in which they are living, and to require his/her attendance at arranged appointments.

Guardianship (section 7) also means that a vulnerable adult can be received into guardianship by the local authority if s/he has a mental illness, severe mental impairment or mental impairment associated with 'abnormally aggressive or seriously irresponsible conduct' or a psychopathic disorder, which results in 'abnormally aggressive or seriously irresponsible conduct'. The guardianship must also be 'necessary in the interests of the welfare of the adult or the protection of other persons'.

Guardianship gives the guardian three basic powers:

- to direct where the adult is to live;
- to require the adult to attend somewhere for the purpose of medical treatment, occupation, education or housing;
- to gain access to the adult at a place in which someone is living.

The Mental Health Act 1983 is currently under review, and further information is outlined in McIver's Chapter 9.

DISCRIMINATORY ABUSE

The Race Relations Act 1976 makes it unlawful for a person to discriminate against another on racial grounds, covering employment, education, facilities, goods, services and premises. The Race Relations Amendment Act 2000 places a general duty on public authorities to have due regard to eradicate unlawful discrimination, and to promote equality of opportunity and good relations between persons of different racial groups, in carrying out their functions.

The Sex Discrimination Act 1975 makes it unlawful to discriminate against a male or female on the grounds of his/her sex.

The Disability Discrimination Act 1995 makes it unlawful to discriminate against a disabled person, and requires employers to make adjustments to arrangements or premises to avoid placing a disabled person at a substantial disadvantage in comparison with non-disabled people.

As from December 2003, discrimination on the grounds of religion or belief and sexual orientation is illegal. Discrimination on the grounds of age is due to become illegal by December 2006.

The Human Rights Act 1998, Schedule 1, article 12, also prohibits discrimination. It states that:

'. . . the enjoyment of the rights and freedoms set forth in the European Convention on Human Rights shall be secured without discrimination on any grounds such as sex, race, colour, language, religion, political or other opinion, national or social origin, association with a national minority, property, birth or other status.'

Another area of concern when working with adults with learning disabilities who may be vulnerable is what may be termed 'institutional abuse'. Section 31 of the Care Standards Act 2000 requires all care homes to be registered with the Commission for Social Care Inspection (CSCI). Where homes are registered, the following may apply:

- if home owners persistently fail to comply with regulations or National Minimum Standards, then registration may be withdrawn and/or they may be prosecuted;
- individuals working in homes may be prosecuted;
- if CSCI officers consider that there is a 'serious risk to the life, health or well being' of residents or patients, then they can obtain an order for the immediate closure of the home (Care Standards Act 2000, section 20);
- specific national minimum standards pertain to care homes for older people; adults aged 18–65, adult placements, domiciliary and nurse agencies.

Concerns regarding the quality of care afforded to adults with learning disabilities are also stated in *Valuing People* (2001b):

'People with learning disabilities are entitled to at least the same level of support and protection from abuse and harm as other citizens. This needs to be provided in a way which respects their own choices and decisions. Good quality services for people with learning disabilities must support them to lead lives safe from harm and abuse, whilst enabling them to lead fulfilling lives.'

(Department of Health 2001b, p. 93)

The law gives carers rights to raise concerns regarding the quality of care. Employed workers have rights to make disclosures as a 'whistleblower', under section 47B of the Employment Rights Act 1996, as an employee she or he:

'. . . has the right not to be subjected to any detriment by any act, or any deliberate failure to act, by his/her employer done on the ground that the worker has made a protected disclosure.'

This therefore protects an employee who discloses information which they reasonably believe tends to show that a criminal offence has been or is likely to be committed; that a person has failed to comply with their legal obligations; or that the health or safety of any individual has been, is being, or is likely to be endangered. Disclosures of such information must be made in good faith.

Section 25 of the Police and Criminal Evidence Act 1984 permits a police officer, where there are reasonable grounds, to make an arrest of someone to prevent him/her from causing physical injury to another person, or to protect a child or other vulnerable adult.

Section 17 outlines the powers to enter and search premises without a warrant, for the purpose of saving a life or limb.

Under common law in England, any person can intervene, without consent, to save life or avoid serious physical harm. This is based on the principle that the action taken by such a person is reasonable and can be professionally justified as immediately necessary for saving life or preventing serious physical harm.

CONSENT

Adults with learning disabilities who are vulnerable need support to ensure that they are not denied the right or opportunity to make their own decisions and give their own consent to lifestyle choices. In English law, no person can give consent on behalf of another (Department of Health 2001a). Where it is necessary, healthcare professionals can and should provide treatment without consent where a person lacks capacity if it is clinically required and is in the best interests of the person. This should only be in exceptional circumstances. However, adults with learning disabilities often find that consent and decisions have been made for them, when they could have been asked or consulted about their own wishes.

Capacity is a legal concept and the Mental Capacity Act 2005 sets out a single, clear test for assessing whether or not a person lacks capacity to make a particular decision at a particular time. It is a 'decision-specific' test, meaning that it needs to be carried out again for other decisions. The act outlines that everything that is being done for a person who lacks capacity must be in that person's best interest. Likewise, it makes it clear that when a vulnerable person who lacks capacity is being cared for, then the person providing the care can do so without inviting legal liability.

VULNERABLE VICTIMS OF CRIME

The Criminal Justice and Court Services Act 2000 requires the National Probation Service to make contact with victims who have experienced a violent or sexual crime, for which the offender received a custodial sentence of a year or more. The purpose is to inform the victim about the sentence, and to establish whether s/he wishes to receive further contact from the Probation Service and whether s/he wishes to be informed when the prisoner is due for release. Research suggests that where these offences have been committed, the victim usually knows the perpetrator, so there may be a higher risk of fear associated with these crimes. It is also known that, in general, adults with learning disabilities are at a much greater risk of having a crime committed against them than within the general public (Brown et al. 1995; Mencap 2001; Williams 1995). Unfortunately, adults with learning disabilities are also less likely to receive justice from the criminal justice system, therefore living in fear of the perpetrator for a substantial period of time. Where cases are prosecuted successfully, there is not the same follow-up afforded to other victims without learning disabilities, and they are often left to their own devices.

Mencap (1999) found that 88 per cent of people with learning disabilities, during a one-year period, had experienced bullying; 53 per cent reported that the bullying continued even when it had been reported. However, Speaking up for Justice (Home Office 1998) has made 78 recommendations that should assist witnesses who are vulnerable or intimidated. Some of these recommendations have been included in the Youth Justice and Criminal Evidence Act 1999. This act defines vulnerable witnesses as:

- witnesses under the age of 17 years at the time of the hearing (section 16(1)(a));
- witnesses suffering from a mental disorder within the meaning of the Mental Health Act 1983 (section 16(2)(a)(i));
- witnesses that have a significant impairment of intelligence and social functioning (section 16(2)(a)(ii)).

Intimidated witnesses are defined as:

- witness is likely to be diminished by reason of fear or distress in connection with testifying in the proceedings (section 17(1)).

The court can order one or more of a range of measures to help the witness in court. These include:

- giving evidence by a live TV link;
- use of an intermediary;
- assistance with communication;
- screens around the witness box to prevent the witness viewing the defendant.

CONCLUSION

As outlined in this chapter, there are a number of laws which can help to support adults with learning disabilities who are vulnerable. However, these will only be effective if carers, students and professionals involved in supporting adults with learning disabilities have an understanding of the various acts, and have the confidence to ensure that ill-treatment, injustice, victimisation and discrimination are tackled. There is current evidence that adults with learning disabilities are bullied, picked on and marginalised by 'mainstream' society, which is evidenced by a recent large-scale survey, as outlined, which states that, for example, 32 per cent of adults with learning disabilities had experienced offensive or rude behaviour because they had learning disabilities (Emerson & Malam 2005). This state of affairs leads to vulnerable adults with learning disabilities depending on carers and professionals to help them to live an 'ordinary life'. This may increase their reliance on others and may decrease their opportunities for independence, placing them potentially 'at risk'.

REFERENCES

Brown, H., Stein, J. & Turk, V. (1995) 'The Sexual Abuse of Adults with Learning Disabilities', *Mental Handicap Research*, **8**: 3–24.

Clare, I. C. H. & Murphy, G. H. (2001) 'Witnesses with Learning Disabilities', *British Journal of Learning Disabilities*, **29**: 79–80.

Department of Health (1989) *Caring for People: Community Care in the Next Decade and Beyond*, London, HMSO.

Department of Health (2000) *No Secrets: Guidance on Developing and Implementing Multi-Agency Policies and Procedures to Protect Vulnerable Adults from Abuse*, London, HMSO.

Department of Health (2001a) *Seeking Consent: Working with People with Learning Disabilities*, London, HMSO.

Department of Health (2001b) *Valuing People: A New Strategy for Learning Disability for the 21st Century*, London, HMSO.

Department of Health (2002) *Protecting the Public: Strengthening Protection against Sex Offenders and Reforming the Law on Sexual Offences*, Cmd 5668, London, HMSO.

Emerson, E. & Malam, S. (2005) *Adults with Learning Difficulties in England 2003/4*, Summary Report, Health and Social Care Information Centre, London, HMSO.

Fearns, D. (2001) 'Learning Disabilities: Recognition and Risk', in B. Littlechild (ed.), *Appropriate Adults and Appropriate Adult Schemes: Service User, Provider and Police Perspectives*, Birmingham, Venture Press.

Goffman, E. (1961) *Asylums: Essays on the Social Situation of Mental Patients and Other Inmates*, Penguin, Harmonsworth.

Harris, J., Allen, D., Cornick, M., Jefferson, A. & Mills, R. (1996) *Physical Interventions: A Policy Framework*, Kidderminster, BILD/NAS.

Home Office (1998) *Speaking up for Justice Report on Vulnerable or Intimidated Witnesses in the Criminal Justice System in England and Wales*, London, HMSO.

Howe Report (1969) *Report of the Committee of Enquiry into Allegations of Ill Treatment of Patients and other Irregularities at the Ely Hospital, Cardiff*, Cmd 3975, London, HMSO.

Jay Committee (1979) *Report of the Committee of Enquiry into Mental Handicap Nursing and Care*, Cmd 7468, London, HMSO.

Mencap (1999) *Living in Fear*, London, Mencap.

Mencap (2001) *Bullying: Living in Fear*, London, Mencap.

O' Brien, J. & Tyne, A. (1989) *The Principle of Normalisation: A Foundation for Effective Services*, London, CMH.

Powell, S. & Northfield, J. (2002) *BILD Factsheets: Physical Interventions*, 20 February, Kidderminster, BILD.

Pringle, I. (2006) *Offences against those with Mental Disorder*, Criminal Law Series, London, Guildhall Chambers, available online at *www.guildhallchambers.co.uk. epoints/Sexual_Offences_Act_2003.html.*

Williams, C. (1995) *Invisible Victims; Crime and Abuse against People with Learning Difficulties*, London, Jessica Kingsley.

Wolfensberger, W. (1972) *The Principle of Normalisation in Human Management Services*, Toronto, National Institute of Mental Retardation.

5 Mental Health Issues and Adults with Learning Disabilities

PAUL MALORET

KEY POINTS

- Issues associated with mental health are highly prevalent in people with learning disabilities; they may often go unrecognised, unreported and, as a result, untreated.
- It is important to make a clear distinction between mental health illness and learning disabilities.
- Adults with learning disabilities can and do experience mental health problems and, indeed, prevalence rates are generally regarded as higher than in the general population.
- When caring for and supporting adults with learning disabilities, it is essential that a grounded understanding of mental health issues is achieved.

INTRODUCTION

This chapter provides an overview of mental health issues and adults with learning disabilities. It identifies areas of the subject in which knowledge is necessary to any professional or informal carers working with people with learning disabilities and associated mental health needs. Priest and Gibbs (2004) suggest that carers of people with learning disabilities are sometimes limited in their understanding of mental health needs and how to adequately assess these needs and provide the required care; this may be the result of deficiency in specific education. The Foundation for People with Learning Disabilities (2005) suggests that there are differences of service provision, depending upon which area of the United Kingdom you live in; also reported is a lack of knowledge about what support is available and how to access it.

It has also been argued that registered nurses working with people with learning disabilities, who themselves are considered as main providers of mental health care to people with learning disabilities, also lack sufficient

Caring for People with Learning Disabilities. Edited by I. Peate and D. Fearns.
Copyright © 2006 by John Wiley & Sons, Ltd.

education in this area. The reality is that mental health needs are highly prevalent in people with learning disabilities, but they can often be unrecognised, unreported and therefore untreated (Northway 2003).

Consideration will be given to how prevalent mental health problems are in learning disabilities and possible reasons for this. It will address how these needs are assessed, how mental health conditions are diagnosed and the carer's role in this process. Subsequent to this, the service provision for mental health needs in people with learning disability will be analysed alongside the interventions that these services may offer.

It is important that from the outset a clear distinction is made, in order to avoid any confusion relating to the differences between mental health and learning disabilities. When people with learning disabilities experience a mental health problem, they are often referred to as having a 'dual diagnosis', which refers to two different conditions co-existing. The two conditions, however, can influence one another; they cannot be viewed as one of the same. This can often be confusing, as aspects of behaviour seen in people with learning disabilities are similar to symptoms of certain mental health conditions and misdiagnosis may result. Care must be taken here, as the term 'dual diagnosis' is not only used in this context, but for other co-existing conditions, namely those who suffer from a mental health condition and misuse a substance, such as alcohol dependency or drug dependency problems.

To examine the difference between learning disabilities and mental health conditions, it is useful to look at definitions of 'mental health' and other terms meaning the same, such as:

- mental illness
- mental disorder
- psychiatric disorder
- mental health problem.

According to the Mental Health Foundation (2003), 'a mental health problem only becomes a serious problem when it interferes with your ability to cope or function on a day to day basis or when your behaviour becomes a concern for others'.

If this were to be considered in the context of people with learning disabilities, it could be argued that some already have 'problems that interfere with their ability to cope or function on a day to day basis'. Also, the behaviour of some people with learning disabilities is certainly of 'a concern for others' and this may not be considered abnormal. A definition from the American Psychiatric Association (1994) helps to clarify this further:

'A mental health problem is a clinically significant behavioral or psychological syndrome or pattern that is associated with present distress or disability or with a significantly increased risk of suffering, death, pain, disability or loss of freedom.'

If we consider this definition in simplistic terms, it can be understood that a mental health problem can be said to exist when there is a change in a person's behaviour, thought processes or mood to the extent that day-to-day life is adversely affected. Therefore, mental health problems are usually temporary, as opposed to a learning disability, which is permanent. People acquire a learning disability before, during or shortly after birth, whereas a mental health problem can occur at any time.

PREVALENCE AND CAUSATION OF MENTAL HEALTH PROBLEMS IN PEOPLE WITH LEARNING DISABILITIES

The mental health needs of people with learning disabilities have only been on the learning disability healthcare agenda for the past 15–20 years. Reid (1994) suggests that historically it was thought that people with learning disabilities did not have the intellectual or cognitive ability to suffer from a mental health disorder. Any noticeable changes in their behaviour were interpreted as part of their learning disability and, on the unusual occasion that signs of mental illness were noted, they were passed on to the local general psychiatric services, as learning disability services were not able to treat them. Reiss (1992) identifies that the issue was in the assessment process, distinguishing whether a 'dual-diagnosed' person's primary need was the learning disability or the mental health problem, i.e. which was more significant to their lives or those around them. Concern was centred on the provision of care, such as whether the patient was to be cared for by those in the mental health or the learning disabilities service. Alongside the responsibility afforded to the appropriate service, funding implications were also an issue. A consequence of labelling psychiatric disorders as secondary often meant funding was also secondary and too often inadequate.

It is now generally agreed that people with learning disabilities can and do experience mental health problems and, indeed, prevalence rates are generally regarded as higher than in the general population. Priest and Gibbs (2004) suggest that their intellectual disability and the cause of this disability, such as prenatal brain damage, make people with learning disabilities susceptible to developing mental health problems. There have been findings of higher prevalence of mental health problems throughout learning disabled populations, i.e. within all levels of cognitive ability and age. Birch et al. (1970) found that 40 per cent of people with learning disabilities suffered from mental illness, compared with 10 per cent of the general population. Stromme and Diseth (2000) found that 33 per cent of people with mild learning disabilities and 42 per cent of those with severe learning disabilities

Table 5.1. Mental illness and learning disabilities (source: Priest & Gibbs 2004)

The highest reported rates of mental illness in learning disabilities fall into four
areas; they are, with the highest reported first:
1. Anxiety disorders
2. Depression
3. Dementia
4. Schizophrenia

suffered from mental illness. Table 5.1 outlines the reported rates of mental
illness in learning disabilities.

ANXIETY DISORDERS

Anxiety disorders are characterised by a persistent and sometimes overwhelming feeling of apprehension, accompanied by a range of physical and
psychological symptoms (Priest & Gibbs 2004). In a lifetime, any given individual has a 5 per cent chance of suffering from an anxiety disorder. Anxiety
disorders are normally considered in several different categories; people with
learning disability are more likely to suffer from three of these, which are
obsessive–compulsive disorder (OCD), generalised anxiety disorder and
panic disorders (American Psychiatric Association 2000).

Anxiety disorders are nearly always related to stress and stressful situations, which can often be the trigger to provoke an attack. Anxiety is a natural
response to stress and only becomes a problem if individuals are unable to
deal with this stress and it has a detrimental effect on a person's ability to
function. Those with learning disabilities are more likely to find themselves
in a greater number of situations that are stressful than people without learning disabilities. This may be a result of not having the skills to deal with these
stressful circumstances adequately, such as paying a water bill or using public
transport – simple procedures that can be very complex if you do not possess
sufficient experience or knowledge (Gates 2003).

Ambelas (1987) ranked 16 life events that can cause severe stress; highly
positioned are moving home, separating of friendships and unemployment.
Gates (2003) suggests people with learning disabilities generally move home
many more times in their lifetime and often do not have a choice of where
they are moving to; they are very often separated from friends as a consequence of moving and most people with learning disabilities have very low
employment opportunities. Additionally, the Foundation for People with
Learning Disabilities (2005) reported that the young people with learning
disabilities interviewed in their research project cited loss and bereavement,
family contact, troubled relationships with peers, social isolation and worries
about specific health conditions as the main contributors to stress and, in turn,
anxiety.

DEPRESSION

Similarly, depression has stress as an influential factor; however, depression is known as 'multifactorial', i.e. it can have a variety of causes. Firstly, there can be a genetic reason, i.e. sufferers may have inherited a genetic make-up from parents or grandparents, which makes them more vulnerable to depression or other mental illnesses. Secondly, there may be a physiological component; a chemical imbalance in the brain is a common factor, i.e. the brain is not producing the correct amount of serotonin, which is a chemical which helps to balance our mood. Thirdly, there may be a psychosocial component, such as bereavement or a challenging social situation. All of these can be a cause on their own or co-exist; the more factors that exist, the more vulnerable a person becomes (Eby & Brown 2005).

DEMENTIA

Dementia is normally a condition associated with older people, in which there is a gradual deterioration in areas such as memory, language and intellect. There will also be changes in mood, behaviour and personality. Alzheimer's disease is known to be the cause for approximately half of all dementias. People with Down syndrome are at a particular risk of developing Alzheimer's disease and it is not exclusive to old age; cases of Alzheimer's disease being diagnosed in people as young as 30 are commonplace in people who suffer from Down syndrome. Prevalence rates of Alzheimer's disease in adults with Down syndrome range from 22 to 45 per cent (Priest & Gibbs 2004).

McCarthy (1997) explains this may be the result of a genetic link between the two conditions, both being linked to chromosome 21, of which Down syndrome sufferers have more than two and thus are more likely to develop Alzheimer's disease. It is also true that people with Down syndrome are living longer today; this may be a result of better provision of healthcare, as people who suffer from Down syndrome are commonly associated with many physical conditions which previously may have been fatal. This increase in age will increase their vulnerability to dementia.

SCHIZOPHRENIA

Pilgrim (2005) describes schizophrenia as a disorder of thinking, perception, mood and behaviour in which the individual loses touch with reality and often experiences impaired function in a range of areas. Classically, people suffering from schizophrenia will experience one or more of the following symptoms:

- Thought disturbance – belief that thoughts and feelings are being taken from their control and others are able to insert new thoughts into their minds.
- Hallucinations – seeing, hearing and smelling objects that are not really there. Sometimes, voices maybe heard that urge them to perform certain acts.
- Delusions – false belief about objects and events, such as *delusions of grandeur*, which describes a person who falsely believes that s/he is royal.

Prevalence of schizophrenia in people with learning disabilities has been reported to be as high as 3 per cent (Deb et al. 2001). This is far higher than that of the general population and when the challenges of assessment are considered later in this chapter, it may appear that this is possibly an under-representation of the actual number of cases. It could be suggested that the cause of schizophrenia lies with an inherited gene, whilst others would disagree and propose that the condition is a product of environmental stress factors, such as sexual abuse and social isolation. Zubin and Spring (1997) suggest that the cause is more likely to be a combination of these factors, i.e. that a biological element exists alongside social and stress factors. An example of this is a person who may have social problems such as being unemployed and/or have financial concerns, or may be suffering from stress caused by bereavement or a life-changing event. Therefore, if an inherited gene existed and that person was subjected to the mentioned stress and social factors, then she or he would be predisposed to developing a mental illness alongside the existing learning disability.

CHALLENGING BEHAVIOUR

Moss et al. (2000) found that there was a strong relationship between mental illness and people with learning disabilities who present 'challenging behaviours' (for a fuller discussion of challenging behaviour, see Chapter 3). Their study showed that mental illness was twice as prevalent in those with challenging behaviours as those without. Depression and anxiety were the most prevalent with those described as having challenging behaviour.

Confusion and fear can often turn into anger and physical aggression. Often, people with a learning disability struggle to cope with events in their lives because they may not possess the insight to realise that situations may, in time, improve. Depression is essentially an over-reaction to loss, whereas anxiety is an over-reaction to the threat of loss. For example, people with learning disabilities may not understand that grieving is a feeling that, given time, may become less overwhelming and they can expect to feel better (Reiss 1992). John's experience helps to demonstrate this.

Case study

John has a mild learning disability and has lived with his mother all his life. When his mother died of cancer John's family felt that he could continue to live in his mother's house, which had been left to him in his mother's will. John continued his life in the house and with his job but, some months later, he started to demonstrate some behavioural changes. His employer said he was notably more irritable and 'moody'; when asked what was wrong, he simply answered 'My mum'. The situation became worse and John stopped turning up for work. His employers called social services and expressed their concerns.

A social worker visited John and reported that the house was in a poor condition, as was John's personal hygiene, i.e. he had not washed or shaved for some weeks. John appeared very anxious and low in mood; the social worker made an urgent referral to the local psychiatric team. John was admitted to hospital and treated on anti-depressant medication; he also received bereavement counselling to help him deal with the loss of his mother.

His counsellor discovered that John had not realised his mother was dead and would not return; he had been told that his mother had gone to heaven; John didn't know where this was and assumed it was a hospital. When she didn't return, he assumed she had left him; he said he felt 'unwanted' and 'missed his mum'. John was diagnosed with depression; his treatment continued over several months, after which time he was discharged and went home. A learning disability nurse was given the responsibility of monitoring John's progress and to observe for any signs of deterioration in his mental health.

John's psychiatrist believed his condition was caused by a number of contributing factors. John's initial reaction to his mother's death was normal but this became abnormal when he was told his mother had 'gone to heaven'; this had given him hope that his mother was coming back. When she did not return, he felt rejected by her; this caused greater sadness and further confusion. Despite this, John attempted to continue with his life, but failed, as he did not possess the coping skills or the practical skills, e.g. housekeeping skills; his previous dependence on his mother and his learning disability had prevented these skills from developing. This frustrated John and made him feel 'helpless' and 'worthless'. John felt he would be a very sad person forever.

It is important to note that people with learning disabilities can suffer from the same mental health problems as anyone else. The four areas chosen here for their high prevalence rates present a higher risk, but people with learning disabilities are certainly represented in other areas, such as mood disorders and personality disorders.

ASSESSMENT AND DIAGNOSES

So far, it has been established that mental health is a major issue for people with learning disabilities and there are a large number of people with learning disabilities who suffer from a variety of mental health conditions. However, the true extent of the problem cannot be known, due to difficulties in assessment, and it is estimated that the actual numbers are far greater than those cited in this chapter. This is largely due to the service users being unable to sufficiently communicate their symptoms; it follows that the more severe the communication problems, the more difficult it is to gain a true assessment. In these circumstances, much of the assessment is reliant upon observations from carers, i.e. changes in behaviour. This presents its own problems, as difficulties arise from differentiating which behaviours are indicative of mental health problems and which are attributed to the symptoms of the person's learning disability (Priest & Gibbs 2004). These problems are demonstrated in the case study of Sarah.

Case study

Sarah, aged 48 years, has a moderate learning disability and very limited communication skills. She is in a community home, where she has lived happily for 15 years. Recently, the care team in the home have been concerned about her behaviour, which appears to be very 'obsessional'. For example, Sarah is spending up to an hour folding her clothes in her wardrobe and she closes doors very slowly and if she is interrupted, she becomes very upset. The staff referred Sarah to the psychiatrist within the local community learning disability team. Sarah attended an outpatient appointment, accompanied by her key worker. The psychiatrist suggested that as Sarah has been previously diagnosed with autism, it is expected for her to have 'routine behaviour' and this would account for her activities. The carers responsible for Sarah took her home; 2 months later, they referred Sarah once more to the team, as her behaviours had increased in frequency and duration. The previous psychiatrist had since left the service and Sarah was seen by another doctor. Her opinion was different and she diagnosed Sarah with obsessional compulsive disorder (OCD). Sarah was prescribed the appropriate medication (normally, an anti-depressant) and asked to return in 6 weeks. By the time of the next appointment, Sarah's behaviours had completely disappeared and the prescribed medication was the only intervention required.

Sarah's poor communication skills provided the psychiatrist with a further barrier in the process of assessment, as much of the process is heavily reliant upon information received from the patient. In the absence of Sarah's ability to communicate her thoughts and emotions, often a third party needs to be involved – someone who knows Sarah well, an example being a family member or a carer. However, this places great importance upon the carer's views and observations; the person providing this information may not have had sufficient education in this area and may omit or misinterpret important information. Often in these circumstances, a psychiatrist will call upon the assistance of a learning disability nurse to help organise a more effective way of observing the patient and completing the assessment process. Wallace (2002) argues that learning disability nurses are receiving more and more referrals for service users with potential mental health problems, but lack sufficient skills to assess them accurately. It appears there are question marks over the abilities of RN's to work with these service users; this problem may well lie with their pre-registration education programmes in learning disability nursing, which are commonly limited concerning aspects of mental health.

The Foundation for People with Learning Disabilities (2005) reported that research conducted to investigate how family carers and care staff identify and respond to changes in the mental and emotional well-being of young people with profound learning disabilities, i.e. those who are assessed as having a very low intellectual ability, found that the majority of the carers were able to identify specific signs that alerted them to changes in emotional and mental well-being and some of the reported symptoms were consistent with psychiatric indicators contained in standard diagnostic instruments.

Accurate diagnosis is important, for several reasons. The nature of the clinical condition is necessary to establish appropriate treatment regimes and any possible causes and risk factors that may require interventions (Hardy & Bouras 2002). In the general population, i.e. people without learning disabilities, mental health problems are largely diagnosed using two diagnostic instruments:

1. ICD-10 – the International Classification of Disorders, section 10, which categorises mental and behavioural disorders; this was published by the World Health Organisation in 1992.
2. DSM-IV – the Diagnostic and Statistical Manual of Mental Disorders, fourth edition, which was published by the American Psychiatric Association, Washington, DC, in 1994.

These and others in use have been applied to people with learning disabilities, but not without difficulty. They often fail to consider behaviours that are attributed to a person's learning disability; altered paths in development are largely based on those who can articulate their feelings. Therefore, in 2001, the Royal College of Psychiatrists published the *Diagnostic Criteria for Psychiatric Disorder for Use with People with Learning Disabilities* (DC-LD) (Royal College of Psychiatrists 2001). This has addressed the above-mentioned problems associated with the generic tools and has given the psychiatrist a greater opportunity for making a correct diagnosis. There are, however, some psychiatrists who still use the older systems and this was the case in Sarah's scenario – errors are not unusual. Even with the DC-LD, inaccuracies occur and it is important to note that the assessment tool is only as good as the person using it.

People with mild learning disabilities, i.e. those whose intellectual abilities range between IQ scores of 50 and 69, are often interviewed as part of the psychiatric assessment process in the same way as people from the general population (Royal College of Psychiatrists 2001). Hardy and Bouras (2002) suggest that with the necessary support and correct approach, people with learning disabilities can generally describe symptoms such as hallucinations, delusions and feelings associated with low mood. However, care must be taken to ensure that the symptoms mentioned by the service users are their own ideas. For example, the author has witnessed such interviews involving service users who are only too happy to answer 'yes' when the assessor makes suggestions about their symptoms; this is because they feel very uncomfortable with the interview and are making attempts to accelerate the process. For people with severe and profound learning disabilities, i.e. those with lower intellectual ability, changes in behaviour and functioning are often the key symptoms and signs of mental illness that their carers need to be aware of (see Table 5.2).

Symptoms outlined in Table 5.2 should be recorded according to frequency, severity, duration and the time of day that these changes occur. It may also be evident that certain factors have an influence and may exacerbate or alleviate such changes, such as a person with obsessional compulsive disorder who becomes very anxious if she or he is prevented from fulfilling a compulsion. It is important to present this information to another healthcare professional in the form of a 'pattern', if indeed one exists. This information can be used to eliminate causes that are not associated with mental health, such as a service user being particularly irritable or even aggressive on a Tuesday; if

Table 5.2. Symptoms and signs that may be associated with mental illness

- Social withdrawal
- Physical appearance, such as changes in pallor, blood-shot eyes
- Sleep pattern, appetite and weight gain or loss
- Loss of skills, such as psychomotor, hand and eye coordination
- Reduction in communication skills
- Onset of or increase in challenging behaviours (not only aggression, but any unusual behaviours)
- Changes in perception of people or environment
- Irritable in mood
- Memory loss
- Changes in energy levels
- Reduced concentration span

this was established, the care team can discover what is different on a Tuesday from any other day. If this pattern in behaviour is not recorded sufficiently, an incorrect decision about a solution could well be the outcome.

Throughout this section, it has been shown that there are many barriers facing both service users and carers in relation to the assessment of mental health needs. Communication methods need to be developed, and the use of non-verbal communication systems may need to be introduced into the assessment process. The following are examples of some techniques used to improve communication and understanding:

- art therapy
- music therapy
- drama therapy
- Makaton, i.e. a sign language designed for use with people with learning disability (Gates 2003).

Additionally, the development of joint working between health and social care professionals and carers needs to be encouraged, to produce meaningful assessments that will assist in correct decisions being made about care packages and diagnosis.

SERVICE PROVISION

People with learning disabilities often have problems accessing generic mental healthcare services; there are many identifiable reasons for this. Within the recent White Paper *Valuing People: A New Strategy for Learning Disability for the 21st Century* (Department of Health 2001), an emphasis has been placed on the mental health needs of people with learning disabilities' being met by generic services with specialist support from learning disability services. Firstly, it is important to establish what is actually meant by 'generic' or 'specialist' services. The terms 'generic' or 'mainstream' refer to those mental health services provided for the whole population, and 'specialist' services refers to services which provide knowledge, skills and expertise to supplement mainstream services where needs cannot be fully met within those generic services. Specialist learning disability services vary across the United Kingdom; however, they would usually consist of assessment and treatment units, community teams consisting of a wide range of disciplines including community learning disability nurses, psychiatrists specialising in learning disabilities, therapists, social workers and psychologists.

The Foundation for People with Learning Disabilities (2002) reported a wide variation in patterns of service delivery for young people with learning disabilities in the United Kingdom. For example, a teenager presenting with a mental health problem could be referred to the local community paediatric service, the child and adolescent mental health service or the learning disability service, depending upon where s/he lived. Generally, generic services will refer to specialist services at the earliest opportunity, if indeed they are available. People with learning disabilities tend to spend time in acute psychiatric services only during times of crisis or when the specialised learning disability teams are unavailable, such as when an admission may be required outside normal hours. Wallace (2002) suggests that mental health nurses do not have the skills or experience to work effectively with people with learning disabilities; this may be due to education in pre-registration programmes for mental health nurses, which are generally not designed to develop these areas of knowledge or skills.

This lack of skills and experience often means that mental health staff are reluctant to offer people with learning disabilities a service; this has an impact on the learning disability services that commonly accept many referrals for people with learning disabilities with mental health issues as their primary need. Wallace (2002) also suggests that this is not ideal either, for the same reason – that learning disability nurses do not have the necessary skills and experience to work effectively with mental health problems. Therefore, it is imperative that both mental health and learning disability services have the appropriate skills, knowledge and experience to be able to support this 'dual-diagnosed' population, to provide a service that addresses the 'whole' person.

In the last 10 years, mental health education has been a high priority for many learning disability care providers, not only within the health service but also within social care and voluntary sector establishments. Many 'dual-diagnosed' service users reside in community homes and are cared for by non-qualified carers; generally, education is purchased for these homes from specialist services or education consultants. Additionally, community nurses from the mental health or learning disability team often support such care homes and advise on issues of care and treatment. For example, if a service user in a community care home has been seen in an outpatients' clinic by a psychiatrist and his/her medication was changed, a community learning disability nurse could help the staff to monitor the effects and/or side effects of this medication. Additionally, the community learning disability team are able to provide or assist with a range of therapeutic interventions.

The question of whether people with learning disabilities and mental health problems should access mainstream generic mental health services or a specialist learning disability service remains unanswered. Certainly, the generic argument can be found in *Valuing People* (Department of Health 2001), which states that specialist support (learning disability services) are more appropriately utilised with 'individuals with significant learning disabilities and mental health problems who cannot be admitted to general psychiatric services'. This would suggest that those whose intellectual disabilities are more severe are more likely to receive a specialist service. *Meeting the Mental*

Health Needs of People with Learning Disabilities (Royal College of Psychiatrists 1996) encourages 'joint working' between the two teams and the specialist service to help and support the generic service, rather than take over the provision of service.

THERAPEUTIC INTERVENTIONS

The term 'therapeutic intervention' refers to a planned action that has the intent to 'heal' or 'cure' (Gates 2003). There are many types of therapeutic interventions that are used to treat mental health problems in people with learning disabilities; generally, they are similar to those for the non-learning disabled population, but some require modification to be successful. Therapies can be used in isolation or with each other; an example of the main therapies used for people with learning disabilities and mental health problems are provided in Table 5.3. It is important to note that many other less well-known types are in use and there are too many to mention in this chapter.

PSYCHOTROPIC MEDICATION

The most prevalent form of intervention remains medication; psychiatric drugs are used in the treatment of all forms of mental illness and there is a strong evidence base to support its appropriate use (Gates 2003; Hardy & Bouras 2002; Pilgrim 2005). There is also evidence to support the use of these drugs for behaviour problems that are not necessarily connected to a mental health problem with people with learning disabilities (Crabbe 1994). For this reason, it is virtually unheard of for a person with a learning disability who presents behaviour difficulties and/or mental health problems not to be on a

Table 5.3. Therapeutic interventions that are commonly used to treat mental health problems in people with learning disabilities

---

Psychotropic medication and interventions and the disorders that they are most likely to be used for:
- anti-psychotic medication – behavioural difficulties and psychosis
- anti-depressant medication – depression
- mood-stabilising agents – bipolar affective disorder
- anxiolytic medication – acute anxiety
- electroconvulsive therapy – severe depression or mania

Psychodynamic interventions and/or psychotherapy may be used to help with:
- behavioural approaches
- cognitive approaches
- counselling

type of medication mentioned in Table 5.3. However, such medication regimes are very often used alongside another type of therapeutic intervention. For example, a service user may have had some anxiety difficulties which seem to have occurred since the death of his mother; a common recommendation would for an introduction to a form of anxiolytic medication to help with the anxiety in the short term and long term for the service user to receive bereavement counselling or a similar psychodynamic intervention. The anxiolytic would help the service user to become relaxed enough to be able to benefit from the counselling sessions. Alternatively, this same service user may be prescribed an anti-depressant to help him overcome his loss; this can also be used in conjunction with counselling and it would not be unusual for these treatments to co-exist.

It is important at this stage to acknowledge differences in terminology used to describe types of medication in the field of psychiatry that, in essence, often refer to the same. Pilgrim (2005) recognises that the psychiatric profession has tended to describe these drugs in relation to their impact on a diagnosed mental disorder, such as anti-depressants for depression and anti-psychotics for psychosis. However, before the Second World War, this was not the case and drugs were seen as 'suppressors of symptoms' and would aim to manage the condition rather than cure it. These were referred to as 'sedatives' or 'tranquilisers', with the most sedating being described as 'major tranquilisers'. The term used today by the medical profession for this group of drugs is 'psychotropic medication'; other names that pertain to a specific type of medication will be discussed under the following subheadings.

ANTI-PSYCHOTIC MEDICATION

Gates (2003) suggests this type of psychotropic medication is used for the following three reasons:

1. The whole range of psychotic illnesses, such as schizophrenia and mania.
2. In the short term, for acute and severe anxiety.
3. Severe self-injurious behaviours and other behavioural difficulties.

The last of these reasons accounts for large numbers of people with learning disabilities being prescribed anti-psychotic medication. Crabbe (1994) suggests that there is an 'overuse' of anti-psychotic medication for this purpose with people with learning disabilities and states that this type of drug intervention is a 'chemical restraint', i.e. the medication is used only to sedate the individual and does not help with the long-term improvement of the behaviour or indeed the cause of it.

Further criticisms are aimed at the many 'side effects' that are common from the use of this type of medication, such as involuntary movements (tremors) of the entire body, uncontrollable eye movements, shuffling gait and blurred vision (Royal College of Psychiatrists 1996). A new generation of anti-psychotics known as atypical anti-psychotics are showing evidence that these side effects are less apparent than they were with the older (typical) anti-psychotics.

ANTI-DEPRESSANT MEDICATION

When used to improve depression, anti-depressant medication is highly effective and research shows that most of the 30 different anti-depressants available in an ever-growing market are very similar in effectiveness (Priest & Gibbs 2004). Anti-depressants are not only effective in treating depressive illnesses, but they are also reported to be effective in other conditions, including:

- anxiety disorders
- phobias
- obsessive–compulsive disorder
- panic disorder
- post-traumatic stress disorder.

In a similar way to the anti-psychotic medications, the side effects reported in the older (tricylic) antidepressants are far fewer in the new serotonin receptor uptake inhibitor (SSRI) versions. It is important and often problematic for people with learning disabilities to understand that the desired effects of the medication will not begin until approximately 2 weeks after the first tablet is taken; this often causes problems with concordance if the results are not obvious immediately. The side effects, however, are normally recognisable immediately, which can help with early determination of suitability for this type of treatment (Pilgrim 2005).

MOOD-STABILISING AGENTS

These are prescribed for the acute treatment and prevention of bipolar affective disorder, previously known as manic depression. This illness was not discussed in the 'Prevalence and causation of mental health problems in people with learning disabilities' section of this chapter, as it is no more prevalent in people with learning disabilities than it is in anyone else. However, this is not to say that it is particularly uncommon within this population and can be extremely difficult to manage when it co-exists with a learning disability. Bipolar affective disorder generally presents as extreme changes in mood that appear in 'cycles' and there are periods of varying states of depression followed often by periods of mania, whereby the sufferer is usually euphoric, irritable, overactive and disinhibited, and may will experience 'grandiose delusions', i.e. they may believe they are Christ or the Queen (Pilgrim 2005).

Priest and Gibbs (2004) suggest that these 'cycles' of mood changes can be more rapid in people with learning disabilities than those of the general population. This causes problems when the most common drug of this type – lithium – is prescribed, as it usually requires a lengthy period of one type of mood to be effective, i.e. the service user needs to be in a manic or hypo-manic stage of the illness for a reasonably lengthy period for the lithium to take effect. Hardy and Bouras (2002) suggest that when lithium cannot be used, anti-epileptic drugs such as carbemazipine and sodium valproate may be useful, as may the newer anti-epileptics such as lamotrigine, for which positive reports of its use in bipolar affective disorder and learning disabilities are becoming commonplace.

ANXIOLYTIC MEDICATION

The Mental Health Foundation (2003) warns that there is a significant risk of addiction to many anxiolytic medications and therefore they should be used in the short term or preferably not at all. However, Priest and Gibbs (2004) propose that diazepam is the most commonly used and can be effective in cases of acute anxiety. Crabbe (1994) advocates the use of diazepam as a pre-medication for the purpose of allaying apprehension before another medi-cation is given or medical procedures that will inevitably cause anxiety; for example, a blood test can be an extremely frightening experience if the patient does not understand the requirement of the procedure and may well perceive the nurse's actions as punitive. Many people with learning disabilities possess phobias of needles, dental examinations, x-rays and other investigative pro-cedures, but very often these intrusive investigations are central to their well-being. Care must be taken in these circumstances, as the administration of a sedating pre-medication can be seen as ethically unsound and will always have implications for consent (Crabbe 1994).

ELECTROCONVULSIVE THERAPY (ECT)

This treatment for severe depression or mania involves passing a mild electri-cal current through the brain, via two electrodes placed on the service user's head. The current induces an epileptic-type seizure lasting for 15–30 seconds; the person will have received a pre-medication which would usually be of the anxiolytic type to help relax the individual beforehand and this is followed by a general anaesthetic, so that the individual is unaware of the procedure in its duration (Cutajar & Wilson 1999). There is little evidence that proves precisely how it works; however, Priest and Gibbs (2004) suggest that its effectiveness in cases of severe depression cannot be doubted. Studies show ECT to be highly effective and faster-acting than all medication (Rogers et al. 1993; Wheeldon et al. 1999).

Cutajar and Wilson (1999) conducted a study on how many people with learning disabilities had received ECT during a 5-year period; they found only eight cases, which is very low in comparison with the general population. This may reflect that ECT requires informed consent, i.e. the recipient must have an understanding of the nature of the treatment, how it works and its long-term effects. ECT is a particularly difficult treatment to explain to depressed patients and when their understanding is further impaired by a learning disability, this task becomes extremely challenging. However, it is not unheard of for service users who are without mental capacity to be forced to receive ECT within the laws set out by the Mental Health Act 1983, but this is rare and only ever considered in extreme circumstances, i.e. after all other treatment for a depressive illness has failed.

PSYCHOLOGICAL INTERVENTIONS/NON-PHYSICAL INTERVENTIONS

These types of interventions do not fall into the traditional medical model that historically has been the way to care for people with mental health needs; there is an explicit taboo on physical contact, which is very different from the previously mentioned interventions. This provides an immediate appeal to the service users, as these types of intervention may be seen as less intrusive. Some 'body therapies' are the exception to this taboo, but any touching is always consented to and must be justifiably therapeutic in its nature; examples would be foot massage in relaxation therapy or compresses in aromatherapy (Grant et al. 2004).

There are many interventions in use of this type and they continue to grow in number and popularity, i.e. in addition to those mentioned within this chapter, good examples are dialectical behaviour therapy (DBT) and early development therapy (EDT), which are held in high regard within mental health (Linehan et al. 1994). It could be argued that the sheer number of options within this field make it very complex for non-therapists to understand and appreciate how they can help and the differences between them. Many health and social care workers within learning disabilities and mental health find this area very confusing, as do the service users themselves. Much of this confusion, again, stems from the multiple terminologies used, much of which, when analysed, have very similar meanings (Gates 2003).

The most well-known psychodynamic interventions are individual or group psychotherapy sessions and, in learning disabilities, these are often manifested in a creative therapy, such as art, drama and music therapy. Psychodynamic treatment methods are directed towards the underlying problem rather than the symptoms. For example, an art therapist receives a referral for a person with severe learning disabilities who has been presenting with some aggressive behaviour; s/he would aim to use the art as a medium to expose the cause of the behaviour. Art, drama and music therapy work very well with all levels of learning disability, but especially with those who have serious communication difficulties (Kuczaj 1994). Hollins (2001) suggests that there are several key areas of difficulty or 'secrets' that people with learning disabilities typically experience, which they are likely to bring to individual or group therapy if given the opportunity. These could be the disability itself, loss, dependency or issues relating to sexuality, to name but a few.

Gates (2003) advocates art therapy's suitability for people with learning disabilities and highlights its flexibility as a major reason for their success. It is 'tailor made' for the service user's individual needs and each intervention is different – typical processes for typical problems do not exist. The pace of the session is dictated by the service user and, more often than not, the sessions are ongoing and only finish if the service user wishes it or the therapy is complete, as opposed to therapy in more generic settings, which it is likely to offer a certain number of sessions only (Gates 2003).

In contrast to psychotherapies, behavioural therapies operate by focusing on the behaviour, rather than its causes, and aim to modify it. Using the same example, if a behavioural therapist received the referral of the person with severe learning disabilities and aggressive behaviour, s/he may not be concentrating on the causes but more on the behaviour itself. However, behaviour therapy in its purest form is largely no longer used. Carers and professionals who have worked within the field of learning disabilities for many years will be very familiar with the terms 'behaviour modification' and 'token economy systems'; these are based upon B. F. Skinner's (1904–90) theory of *operant conditioning*, which can be described as learning by consequences. The aim is to increase desirable behaviour through manipulating the consequences of that behaviour. Positive reinforcements for desirable behaviour exist alongside negative reinforcements to undesirable behaviours; it is the negative reinforcements that would too often carry punitive measures which have seen this form of intervention largely discredited in today's practice. An example would be that when a service user with destructive behaviour broke a piece of furniture, she or he would have a favourite item taken away from him/her. The general consensus appears to be that good practice involves practitioners' rewarding good behaviour, but not punishing poor behaviour (Hollins 2001).

There are more recently developed interventions that adopt the behavioural model, such as relaxation therapy and anger management therapy; these have cognitive as well as behavioural components. Cognitive approaches are based on the idea that mental health problems are caused by problems in the way we think. In other words, how we think determines how we feel; therefore, cognitive therapy addresses an individual's negative thoughts and beliefs. It has been shown to be very successful with mental health problems, especially depression; some would argue that it is as effective as medication (Grant et al. 2004).

Contemporary practice suggests that behavioural and cognitive approaches are used concurrently and the most frequently used is cognitive–behaviour therapy (CBT). It is important to clarify that CBT is not a single therapy but is more of an umbrella term for many different therapies, of which the number seems to grow continuously. Priest and Gibbs (2004) indicate that its significance within mental health stems from its ability to deal with both the symptoms and the behaviour. CBT aims to confront negative feelings and reform them in a more positive light. An example would be a service user struggling to come to terms with a bereavement; the CBT therapist may aim to move the thoughts of negativity such as 'I miss them' or 'I need them' to 'We had some great times together'. However, CBT requires the ability to understand the reasoning behind the changes in thinking and articulate those thoughts so that service users can work together with the therapist; it is argued that without this insight, it cannot be successful, i.e. people with learning disabilities or psychotic patients may find this intervention fairly limited in its achievement. Similarly, the problems of poor communication with people with learning disabilities can hinder the effectiveness of counselling; however, given the correct environment and a skilled counsellor, people with learning disabilities are shown to develop emotionally with its help. Clarke (1994) suggests that the root of counselling is the principle that all human beings seek to grow, develop, expand, maintain and restore themselves. It is therefore the prime task of the therapist to create those conditions which will be conducive to their growth. The approach must be person-centred and relies on a genuine and unconditional acceptance of the service user.

CONCLUSION

Associated mental health problems and people with learning disabilities is an area that has attracted vast amounts of research and opinion in recent years; consequentially, there are varying degrees of reliability and validity in this work and there are, at times, blatant contradictions and disagreements. This chapter has been an attempt to summarise much of this information and present it in a comprehensible manner. When working with people with learning disabilities, it is essential that a grounded understanding of mental health issues is achieved because, more often than not, it is the responsibility of the carer to ensure that such needs are reported and met. The observations of a carer who knows the personality of a service user well are invaluable; this shared information from an individual who possesses some knowledge of mental health is more valuable still.

It is, however, unrealistic to know everything about a vast area of health care such as this without extensive further study and the knowledge shared in this chapter is merely the tip of the iceberg. Additionally, the facts presented in this chapter commonly affect people with learning disabilities; it is important to note that other areas of assessment, treatment and diagnosis are not exclusive to those without learning disabilities and each scenario must at all times be individually assessed. Because of some of the problems of assessing people with learning disabilities already highlighted in this chapter, people may make too many assumptions and decisions about care and treatment. Hasty decisions can be dangerously incorrect; it is far better to be deliberate and methodical in your approach as opposed to reactionary and risk inaccuracies.

REFERENCES

Ambelas, A. (1987) 'Life Events and Mania: A Special Relationship?', *British Journal of Psychiatry*, **150**: 135–246.

American Psychiatric Association (1994) *Diagnostic and Statistical Manual of Mental Disorders – DSM-IV*, Washington, American Psychiatric Association.

American Psychiatric Association (2000) *Diagnostic and Statistical Manual of Mental Disorders – DSM-IV-TR (Text Revised)*, Washington, American Psychiatric Association.

Birch, H., Richardson, S. & Baird, D. (1970) *Mental Subnormality in the Community: A Clinical and Epidemiological Study*, Baltimore, Williams and Wilkinson.

Clarke, P. T. (1994) 'A Person Centred Approach to Stress Management', *British Journal of Guidance and Counselling*, **22**(1): 27–37.

Crabbe, H. F. (1994) 'Pharmacotherapy in Mental Retardation', in N. Bouras (ed.), *Mental Health in Mental Retardation: Recent Advances and Practices*, Cambridge, Cambridge University Press.

Cutajar, P. & Wilson, D. (1999) 'The Use of ECT in Intellectual Disability', *Journal of Intellectual Disability Research*, **43**(5): 421–7.

Deb, S., Matthews, T. & Holt, G. (2001) *Practice Guidelines for the Assessment and Diagnoses of Mental Health Problems in Adults with Intellectual Disability*, Brighton, Pavilion.

Department of Health (2001) *Valuing People: A New Strategy for Learning Disability for the 21st Century*, London, Department of Health.

Eby, L. & Brown, N. (2005) *Mental Health Nursing Care*, Englewood Cliffs, NJ, Prentice Hall.

Foundations for People with Learning Disabilities (2002) *Count Us In: The Report of The Committee of Inquiry into Meeting the Mental Health Needs of Young People with Learning Disabilities*, London, Mental Health Foundation.

Foundations for People with Learning Disabilities (2005) *Making Us Count: Identifying and Improving Mental Health Support for Young People with Learning Disabilities*, London, Mental Health Foundation.

Gates, B. (2003) *Learning Disabilities: Towards Inclusion*, London, Churchill Livingstone.

Grant, A., Mills, J., Mulhern, R. & Short, N. (2004) *Cognitive Behaviour Therapy in Mental Health Care*, London, Sage.

Hardy, S. & Bouras, N. (2002) 'The Presentation and Assessment of Mental Health Problems in People with Learning Disabilities', *Learning Disability Practice*, **5**(3): 33–9.

Hollins, S. (2001) 'Psychotherapeutic Methods', in A. Dosen & K. Day (eds), *Treating Mental Illness and Behavior Disorders in Children and Adults with Mental Retardation*, Washington, American Psychiatric Press.

Kuczaj, E. (1994) 'Art Therapy and Learning Disability', *Mencapnews*, London, Mencap.

Linehan, M., Tutch, D., Heard, H. & Armstrong, H. (1994) 'Interpersonal Outcome of Cognitive Behavioural Treatment for Chronically Suicidal Borderline Patients', *Journal of Psychiatry*, **151**: 1771–6.

McCarthy, J. M. (1997) 'Ageing and Learning Disabilities', in S. Read (ed.), *Psychiatry in Learning Disability*, London, WB Saunders, pp. 237–53.

Mental Health Foundation (2003) *Mental Health Problems: A Fact Sheet*, available online at *http://www.mentalhealth.org.uk* (accessed 26 February 2006).

Moss, S., Emerson, E. & Kiernan, C. (2000) 'Psychiatric Symptoms in Adults with Learning Disabilities and Challenging Behaviour', *British Journal of Psychiatry*, **177**: 453–6.

Northway, R. (2003) 'Foreword', in H. Priest & G. Gibbs (eds), *Mental Health Care for People with Learning Disabilities*, London, Churchill Livingstone, pp. 1–17.

Pilgrim, D. (2005) *Key Concepts in Mental Health*, London, Sage Publications.

Priest, H. & Gibbs, M. (2004) *Mental Health Care for People with Learning Disabilities*, London, Churchill Livingstone.

Reid, A. (1994) 'Psychiatry and Learning Disabilities', *British Journal of Psychiatry*, **164**(5): 613–17.

Reiss, S. (1992) 'Assessment of a Man with Dual Diagnosis', *Mental Retardation*, **30**: 1–16.

Rogers, A., Pilgrim, D. & Lacey, R. (1993) *Experiencing Psychiatry: User Views of Services*, Basingstoke, MIND.

Royal College of Psychiatrists (1996) *Meeting the Mental Health Needs of People with Learning Disabilities*, London, Royal College of Psychiatrists.

Royal College of Psychiatrists (2001) *DC-LD (Diagnostic Criteria for Psychiatric Disorder for Use with Adults with Learning Disabilities/Mental Retardation)*, Occasional Paper OP48, London, Gaskill.

Stromme, P. & Diseth, T. H. (2000) 'Prevalence of Psychiatric Diagnoses in Children with Mental Retardation: Data from a Population-Based Study', *Developmental Medicine and Child Neurology*, **42**: 266–70.

Wallace, B. (2002) 'Boxed in: The Challenge of Dual Diagnoses', *Learning Disability Practice*, **5**(3): 24–6.

Wheeldon, T. J., Robertson, C., Eagles, J. M. & Reid, I. (1999) 'The Views and Outcomes of Consenting and Non-Consenting Patients Receiving ECT', *Psychological Medicine*, **29**: 221–3.

Zubin, J. & Spring, B. (1997) 'Vulnerability: A New View of Schizophrenia', *Journal of Abnormal Psychology*, **86**: 103–26.

6 Epilepsy and Adults with Learning Disabilities

DEBRA FEARNS

KEY POINTS

- Approximately 1000 people die every year as a result of epilepsy, mostly as a result of seizures.
- Epilepsy is the most common neurological disorder, affecting people of all ages. At least one in 20 people will have one seizure during their lifetime.
- Accurate eye-witness accounts are fundamental in helping to make a correct diagnosis, as, often, the person having the seizure has no recollection of what has happened.
- The risk of premature death in adults with a learning disability with epilepsy is two to three times greater than in the general population.

INTRODUCTION

This chapter will examine epilepsy and the implications of identification, types of seizures, prevalence and the care of epilepsy in adults with learning disabilities. Epilepsy will be defined and the categories of epilepsy will be outlined. The management of epilepsy will be examined and strategies discussed. The use of anti-epileptic drugs (AEDs) will be examined in the context of recently published National Institute for Health and Clinical Excellence (NICE) Guidelines (2004). Epilepsy is still a stigmatising condition and, due to its unpredictable pattern, can cause fear and distress in those who do not understand what may be happening to a person having a seizure. Betts and Smith (1994) also point out that people with epilepsy are neglected in comparison with people, for example, who have diabetes or asthma. It must be noted that epilepsy is not a benevolent condition; approximately 1000 people die every year as a result of epilepsy, mostly as a result of seizures (Hanna et al. 2002).

Caring for People with Learning Disabilities. Edited by I. Peate and D. Fearns.
Copyright © 2006 by John Wiley & Sons, Ltd.

Epilepsy can be defined as:

'. . . a tendency to have recurrent seizures, brought about by a sudden, temporary interruption in some or all of the neurones in the brain.'

(National Society for Epilepsy)

PREVALENCE

One single seizure does not constitute epilepsy. The term 'epilepsy' may be properly used if an adult has a tendency to experience repeated seizures due to an intrinsic disturbance of neuronal functions within the brain. However, it must be noted that epilepsy is not a single condition, and it will affect people in different ways. Epilepsy is the most common neurological disorder, affecting people of all ages. At least one in 20 people will have one seizure during their lifetime:

'At any one time between 1 in 140 and 1 in 200 people in the UK (at least 300,000 people) are being treated for epilepsy. In an average PCT (Primary Care Trust) of 150,000 people, between 75 and 120 will develop epilepsy each year.'

(Clinical Effectiveness Group 2003)

Nonetheless, epilepsy rates and prevalence are much higher amongst adults with learning disabilities. The Department of Health (2001) point out, for example, that the prevalence of epilepsy in adults who have a mild learning disability is 10 times greater than in the general population, i.e. 5 per cent. Having a learning disability does not cause epilepsy, nor does having epilepsy cause learning disabilities. However, both epilepsy and learning disabilities may be due to fundamental brain damage existing from birth or as a result of infection or head injury, hence explaining this higher incidence. Stokes et al. (2004) indicate that a general practitioner (GP) with 2000 patients will typically have 36 patients who have learning disabilities, and six of those will have severe learning disabilities. McVicker et al. (1994) believe that adults with Down's syndrome have a higher rate of epilepsy as they age, with 46 per cent aged over 50 having epilepsy. These figures are broadly replicated by the Department of Health (2001):

'The rate of "active" epilepsy for people with mild or moderate learning disabilities is 5% compared to a normal rate of 0.5% in the general population. We may expect to find 30% of people with severe learning disabilities at risk of developing epilepsy, rising to 50% amongst those with profound learning disabilities. The condition originates in childhood for the majority. For people with Down's syndrome the onset of seizures in middle age may be associated with the onset of dementia.'

(Department of Health 2001, p. 101)

CAUSES OF EPILEPSY

Any person's brain has the capacity to produce a seizure, if the circumstances are right; however, most brains are unlikely to do this spontaneously. It can therefore be said that the majority of people have a high 'seizure threshold'. Therefore, a person with a low 'seizure threshold' may be at risk of developing epilepsy spontaneously, without other factors necessarily being involved. A person's 'seizure threshold' may be lowered if the brain is subject to injury, or to unusual stimulation. If the brain injury is severe, following a road traffic accident, birth trauma, tumour, infection or a stroke for example, epilepsy may develop as a consequence. Stokes et al. (2004) indicate higher prevalence rates in some adults – 75 per cent, for example, in adults with cerebral palsy or brain damage. Adults with Down's syndrome and those with other chromosomal disorders often have epilepsy, and seizure frequency may increase as they age, alongside an increase in Alzheimer's disease. Occasionally, a pattern of predisposition can be seen in families, if several members have epilepsy, but the genetics of epilepsy are very complex, so it cannot be stated with certainty.

DIAGNOSING EPILEPSY

Epilepsy diagnosis is not based on a single, 'one-off' seizure, but on the history of more than one epileptic seizure. A GP should refer patients who have seizures to the relevant specialists. A neurologist or other epilepsy specialist will confirm a diagnosis of epilepsy. These specialists are called 'epileptologists'. They may be neurologists or neuropsychiatrists who have additional training and expertise in epilepsy. Accurate eye-witness accounts are fundamental in helping to make a correct diagnosis, as, often, the person having the seizure has no recollection of what has happened. This history is the foundation of epilepsy diagnosis. Other investigations may provide additional information about the person's general health and well-being, but they do not confirm the diagnosis. Blood tests, for example, check out a person's general health, and may help to exclude a metabolic cause for the seizures. An electroencephalogram (EEG) measures the electrical activity of the brain, but should not be routinely used to exclude a diagnosis of epilepsy. However, an EEG may be of relevance in helping to classify the types of epileptic seizures that the person is having (National Society for Epilepsy 2003).

Accurate diagnosis may rely on a number of factors; however, it is important, as carers, to be aware of useful steps that can be taken to support a diagnosis in adults with learning disabilities:

- 'Keep written accounts/notes of what happened to the person before, during and after the seizure.

- Refer to the person's GP, so a full medical assessment may be made as quickly as possible after the seizure.
- Ask the GP to refer the person on to an epilepsy specialist.
- Observe the person closely after his/her seizure.
- Keep written records, particularly of subsequent seizures.'

(Epilepsy Connections 2004)

CATEGORIES OF EPILEPSY

IDIOPATHIC EPILEPSY

This is used to categorise epilepsy where there is no clear environmental cause. It is therefore presumed that genetic factors predominate. There are often no other disabilities present, and the response to drug treatment is usually very good.

SYMPTOMATIC EPILEPSY

This occurs usually as a result of some kind of structural abnormality in the brain. This may have been present from birth, or may occur later in life. It is possible that other disabilities may also be present, caused by the same abnormality. Response to drug treatment may be variable.

DEFINITION OF A SEIZURE

A seizure happens when ordinary, highly complex brain activity is suddenly disrupted, and can take many forms.

CLASSIFICATION OF SEIZURES

All classifications are based on the international classification of seizures (Dreifuss 1989).

GENERALISED SEIZURES

Tonic–clonic (previously known as 'grand mal')

The person becomes rigid, and may fall if standing. The muscles relax and then tighten rhythmically, causing the person to convulse. The breathing becomes laboured and the person may also become incontinent. There is a brief period of unconsciousness and, on waking, the person may be tired and confused and have a headache.

Tonic

The person is affected by generalised stiffening of muscles, without rhythmical jerking.

Atonic (drop attacks)

This consists of a sudden loss of muscle tone. The person may fall to the floor, suddenly, without warning.

Myoclonic

The person experiences abrupt jerking of the limbs. This type of seizure often happens within a short time of the person waking up.

Absences

These consist of a brief interruption of consciousness without any other signs, except possibly a fluttering of the eyelids. It commonly occurs in children, and was previously known as 'petit mal'. These 'absences' may be mistaken for 'daydreaming' by the person so affected (NICE Health Technology Appraisal 2004).

PARTIAL (OR FOCAL SEIZURES)

Simple partial

In this instance, the person's consciousness is not impaired, and seizures are usually confined to rhythmical twitching of one limb, or part of a limb, or to unusual tastes or sensations such as pins and needles in a distinct part of the body. Sometimes, they may also be referred to as a 'warnings' or 'auras', as they may develop into other sorts of seizures.

Complex partial

The person's consciousness is affected. Seizures may then be characterised by a change in awareness, as well as 'semi-purposive' movements, such as fiddling with clothes or nearby objects.

Status epilepticus

This has been defined as a condition in which epileptic activity persists for over 30 minutes' duration. This is a medical emergency, and requires immediate intervention. Emergency treatment should, however, be started once a seizure has persisted, or there are serial seizures for more than 5 minutes. Management is as follows:

- Call the emergency services.
- Secure airway.
- Give oxygen (if possible).
- Assess cardiac and respiratory function.
- Give the person their emergency AED, e.g. rectal diazepam.
- Continually monitor the person's condition.

(Clinical Effectiveness Group 2003)

Stokes et al. (2004) have published guidelines for treating status epilepticus in adults and children, primarily to improve the treatment of people in status epilepticus, once admitted to hospital.

STEPS TO TAKE WHEN AN ADULT HAS A SEIZURE

Simple partial seizure:

- Steer the person away from any pressing dangers.
- Offer support and comfort to the person.
- Stay until the person recovers, in case she or he has a tonic–clonic seizure.

Complex partial seizures:

- Steer the person away from any pressing dangers.
- Do not confine or try to divert the person.
- Stay with the person until she or he recovers.

Absence seizures:

- Steer the person away from any pressing dangers.
- Confirm that she or he has not missed any vital information during an 'absence'.

Tonic, atonic and myoclonic seizures:

- Make sure the person has no injuries, and, where necessary, give first aid.
- Stay until the person recovers and offer support and comfort.

(Epilepsy Connections 2004)

ANTI-EPILEPTIC DRUGS

Anti-epileptic drugs (AEDs) are the preference for the treatment of epilepsy. These AEDs will control seizures for most people with epilepsy, but there will be a minority of people for whom these AEDs are less effective. AEDs are effective in stabilising the electrical brain activity that causes seizures, particularly if the cause is idiopathic. AEDs do not provide a cure for epilepsy, but enable the majority of people to live without the fear of having seizures.

As a student or carer of an adult with learning disabilities who has epilepsy, it is essential that you familiarise yourself with the AEDs used by the adult with a learning disability whom you are caring for. All drugs or medications have two names: the 'generic' name, which is the drug's 'chemical' name, and its 'brand' name, which the drug manufacturer gives it. For example, carbamazepine is the generic name, and its brand name is Tegretol. However, you must ensure that the adult whom you are supporting always takes the same 'brand' of drug, as there may be subtle differences in the way in which drugs are prepared by different manufacturers, and this could have an effect on their effectiveness in controlling seizures.

AEDs work to prevent the abnormal electrical activity that triggers seizures. AEDs are absorbed into the bloodstream and transported to the brain. AEDs need to remain at a constant level in the bloodstream throughout a 24-hour period, and therefore AED levels need to be maintained. This means that AEDs should be taken at the same time every day, at the same dose, to maintain this delicate balance, as too little or too much of the drug can result in more seizures occurring. Some AEDs are taken only once per day, as this helps to maintain a constant level throughout the day and night (Epilepsy Scotland 2005).

AEDs affect the brain in different ways, therefore, some AEDs are more effective for some types of epilepsy than others. As a student or carer, you need to make yourself aware of the type(s) of seizure that the service users have and the side effects of the AEDs that they are taking. This is so that you can monitor and identify any potential side effects of the AEDs and ensure that any other factors relevant to their health status are noted and acted on, if necessary.

An epilepsy specialist should ensure that each adult with epilepsy has an individualised AED treatment plan that is based on the type(s) of seizure pattern, other associated health problems and other medication she or he may be taking. The first consideration should be that the person is started on one AED (monotherapy). Only if this fails to work adequately should another drug be tried. Stokes et al. (2004) state that 'If an AED has failed because of adverse effects or continued seizures, a second drug should be started (which may be an alternative first-line or second-line drug) and built up to an adequate or maximum tolerated dose and then the first drug should be tapered off slowly' (Stokes et al. 2004, p. 56). Combination therapy (more than one AED) 'should only be considered when attempts at mono-therapy with AEDs have not resulted in seizure freedom' (Stokes et al. 2004, p. 56).

During the past 12 years, newer AEDs have been introduced to supplement more established AEDs, such as sodium valporate (Epilim), phenytoin (Epanutin) and carbamazepine (Tegretol). Newer AEDs include lamotrigine (Lamictal), levetiracetam (Keppra), tiagabine (Gabitril) and gabapentin (Neurontin), amongst others. These newer AEDs are suggested for treatment where other AEDs have not benefited the person in controlling seizures. However, newer AEDs may not be more effective in controlling seizures, despite hopes that they will improve the quality of life for people with epilepsy. Indeed, the National Institute for Clinical Excellence (NICE) (2004) recommends that the first-line treatment of epilepsy in adults should continue to be based on established medications such as sodium valporate. This NICE report states that these newer epilepsy drugs do not improve seizure control or quality of life when compared with the standard treatments (sodium valporate or carbamazepine). It concludes that the newer AEDs should only be used when more established standard treatments are unsuitable or unsuccessful in managing seizures. The NICE Health Technology Appraisal (2004) reviewed the evidence and they based their advice on both the clinical effectiveness and the cost of drugs reviewed for the treatment of epilepsy in adults.

It is essential that AEDs are monitored, and that the person who has epilepsy is started on the lowest possible dose. The purpose of this is twofold: firstly, it will help to lessen potential side effects; secondly, the rate at which the dosage of the AED is increased will help the epileptologist decide on an appropriate dose that provides the maximum control of seizures with the fewest side effects. Monotherapy is the preferred approach to treatment with AEDs (NICE Health Technology Appraisal 2004).

Many adults with moderate and severe learning disabilities may have other associated health conditions (co-morbidity) which could be a complicating factor both in diagnosing epilepsy, but also in ensuring that AEDs do not interact with any other medication that they may be taking for their health condition. As the carer or student, you will need to help the service users to self-monitor or monitor on their behalf any side effects from the AED and any other medication. The range of side effects varies, depending on the AED being used. For example, possible side effects of carbamazepine include blurred or double vision, headaches, drowsiness and skin rashes. In addition, for women, rarely, there may be foetal abnormalities (British Medical Association and the Royal Pharmaceutical Society 2005). Many AEDs also cause some weight gain, and therefore you need to help adults with learning disabilities to maintain a healthy diet, as obesity can be a problem for adults with learning disabilities (Wood 1994).

Regular monitoring should help to identify both changes in the degree or severity of side effects and an increase in seizure activity, necessitating changes in the AED dosage until maximum control is achieved. As the carer or student, you may need to ensure that the service user takes the AED at regular intervals, to maintain the AED in the bloodstream. If a service user misses a dose, advice *must* be sought from the epileptologist as to the best course of action, if it is not already outlined in his/her care plan. It is also important to note that service users need to continue taking AEDs *until* the epileptologist outlines a supervised withdrawal, where this may be appropriate (Epilepsy Scotland 2005).

WOMEN AND AEDS

There are particular considerations that need to be taken into account when supporting women with learning disabilities who have epilepsy. Women with learning disabilities should not be excluded from the same services available to all women, but information may need to be modified in order to meet their needs. The issue of contraception needs to be considered carefully with women of child-bearing age.

Non-hormonal contraception methods have no side effects for women with epilepsy. It needs to be noted that hormonal contraception methods, such as the contraceptive pill, may affect the usefulness of the AEDs. This is primarily because of the interaction of female hormones with AEDs. AEDs such as sodium valporate and newer AEDs lamotrigine and levetiracetam do not impact on the effectiveness of hormonal contraceptives. However, carbamazepine, phenobarbitone, phenytoin, primidone and ethosuximide do reduce the effectiveness of hormonal contraceptives. These issues need to be discussed with both the epileptologist and the woman's GP (Royal Society of Medicine 2004).

Women with mild learning disabilities and epilepsy need to be offered advice about pregnancy, preferably before becoming pregnant, in the same way as other women with epilepsy. These issues should be discussed at every annual review of epilepsy (or when the woman's condition dictates) while the woman is of child-bearing age. Where pregnancy occurs, the woman will still need to continue taking AEDs, although adjustments to the dosage may be made by the epileptologist. The danger to the mother and baby from not taking AEDs and having seizures is usually greater than that associated with taking AEDs (British Medical Association and the Royal Pharmaceutical Society 2005; NICE Guidelines 2004).

Further detailed guidance on the management of pregnancy, labour and caring for the baby can be found in *Primary Care Guidelines for the Management of Females with Epilepsy* (October 2004), and from the National Society for Epilepsy website. Additional guidance has been issued by Stokes et al. (2004).

MONITORING EPILEPSY IN ADULTS WITH LEARNING DISABILITIES

As carers and students, it is important to have an understanding of the service users whom you are working with. This includes understanding the seizures that the service user has, which may be of more than one type. This will help you to identify the best course of action and treatment for the service user. In addition, you need to be aware that symptoms can vary over a period of time, and you should make allowances for this.

It is very important that accurate accounts of seizure activity are recorded for monitoring purposes. This recording should identify key factors that should include the following points:

- What were the time and date of the seizure?
- What was the service user doing before the seizure?
- Was the service user awake or sleeping?
- Were there any trigger factors?
- Did you notice anything unusual about the service user before the seizure?
- Can the service user recall any unusual sensation before the seizure?
- What exactly was the first thing that happened?
- Can you describe the events?
- How long did each stage of the seizure last?
- Was there evidence of change in tone or abnormal movements?
- Did the service user lose consciousness?
- Did you notice alterations in the service user's level of awareness?
- Did the service user become incontinent of bladder or bowel?
- Has the service user sustained any injuries due to the seizure?
- How did the seizure end?
- What was the service user like afterwards and subsequently?
- Did the service user have any after-effects?

(Adapted from Enlighten – Tackling Epilepsy 2004)

As well as recording the seizure in writing, with adults with severe learning disabilities and epilepsy, video recordings can also aid the eye witness account so that an accurate picture is presented (Stokes et al. 2004). Monitoring seizures is essential and will help the service users to manage their seizures so that they can enjoy a good quality of life.

CARE OF THE PERSON WITH EPILEPSY

Epilepsy services have been criticised for not providing appropriate, high-quality care, with services portrayed as having little direction and ineffective communication channels between primary and secondary care (Ridsdale 2000). In addition, the Department of Health has recently published its Health Action Plan, *Improving Services for People with Epilepsy* (Department of Health 2003). This was in response to Hanna et al.'s (2002) report on epilepsy-related deaths. Hanna et al. (2002) report that the risk of premature death in adults with epilepsy is two to three times greater than in the general population.

The Action Plan has three main targets for improvement:

• care, management and treatment of epilepsy
• information provision
• pathology and post-mortem investigations.

Hanna et al. (2002) reported that 54 per cent of all adults were receiving poor and inadequate care. Of these, 20 per cent had inadequate AED management, 5 per cent had no evidence of a care package and 6 per cent of adults with learning disabilities were 'lost' in the transition from child to adult services. They also reported poor communication between healthcare professionals and reported that only 10 per cent of families were contacted by a specialist after an epilepsy-related death.

Learning-disability specialists, students and carers all need to increase their awareness of the higher risk of death for people with learning disabilities and epilepsy. Stokes et al. (2004) indicate that all adults with learning disabilities and epilepsy should have a comprehensive risk-assessment package. They suggest that it should include:

• bathing and showering
• preparing food
• using electrical equipment
• managing prolonged or serial seizures
• the impact of epilepsy in social settings
• SUDEP*
• the suitability of independent living, where the rights of the individual are balanced with the role of the carer.

(*SUDEP: Sudden Unexpected Death in Epilepsy)

(Stokes et al. 2004, p. 326)

Every adult with a learning disability and epilepsy should be reviewed annually (or sooner if the person's health condition dictates) by an epileptologist, to ensure that treatment regimes are appropriate and helpful in the management and control of seizures.

CONCLUSION

Epilepsy is the most common neurological disorder, affecting people of all ages, with a prevalence rate of 0.5 per cent in the general population (National Society for Epilepsy 2003). However, in the learning disability population, this rises to 5 per cent of people with mild or moderate learning disabilities, and up to 50 per cent amongst those with profound learning disabilities (Department of Health 2001). Services have not always been responsive to the needs of adults with learning disabilities and epilepsy, but this needs to change, as all 'people with learning disabilities are entitled to have access to specialist clinics, including tertiary services' (Department of Health 2001, p. 101). Effective monitoring of AEDs will provide a better quality of life for the service user, and, as students and carers, you need to have a greater understanding of how epilepsy is affecting the service user and be responsive to subtle changes indicating changes in his or her health status. Accurate monitoring and recording are essential skills that you need to develop to help deliver high-quality care.

REFERENCES

Betts, T. & Smith, K. (1994) 'New Departures in Epilepsy Care: An Epilepsy Liaison Service', *Seizure*, **3**: 301–8.

British Medical Association and the Royal Pharmaceutical Society (2005) *British National Formulary*, London.

Clinical Effectiveness Group (2003) *Fast-Track Summary Guidelines*, London, Department of General Practice and Primary Care, Barts and the London Queen Mary's School of Medicine and Dentistry.

Department of Health (2001) *Valuing People: A New Strategy for Learning Disability for the 21st Century*, Cm 5056, London, HMSO.

Department of Health (2003) *Improving Services for People with Epilepsy*, 30768, London, HMSO.

Dreifuss, F. E. (1989) 'Classification of Epileptic Seizures and the Epilepsies', *Pediatric Clinics of North America*, **36**: 265–79.

Enlighten – Tackling Epilepsy (2004), Fact sheet 6, *How to Record Seizures*, Edinburgh.

Epilepsy Connections (2004) *Leaflet 3: Recording Seizures*, London, Epilepsy Research Foundation, available online at *www.erf.org.uk*.

Epilepsy Scotland (2005) *Treatment Fact Sheet, 2005*, Glasgow, Epilepsy Scotland.

Hanna, N. J., Black, M., Sander, J. W., Smithson, W. H., Appleton, R., Brown, S. & Fish, D. R. (2002) *Epilepsy: Death in the Shadows*, National Sentinel, National Clinical Audit of Epilepsy Related Deaths, London, The Stationery Office.

McVicker R. W., Shanks O. E. & McClelland R. J. (1994) 'Prevalence and Associated Features of Epilepsy in Adults with Down's Syndrome', *British Journal of Psychiatry*, **164**: 528–32.

National Institute for Clinical Evidence (2004), *Newer Drugs for Epilepsy in Adults*, Technology Appraisal 76, London, National Institute for Clinical Excellence.

National Society for Epilepsy (2003) *Clinical Effectiveness Guidelines*.

NICE Guidelines (2004) *The Epilepsies: The Diagnosis and Management of the Epilepsies in Adults and Children in Primary and Secondary Care*, London, National Institute for Clinical Excellence.

Ridsdale, L. (2000) 'The Effect of Specially Trained Epilepsy Nurses in Primary Care: A Review', *Seizure*, **9**: 43–6.

Royal Society of Medicine (2004) *Primary Care Guidelines for the Management of Females with Epilepsy*, London, Royal Society of Medicine Press.

Stokes, T., Shaw, E. J., Juarez-Garcia, A., Camosso-Stefinovic, J. & Baker, R. (2004) *Clinical Guidelines and Evidence Review for the Epilepsies: Diagnosis and Management in Adults and Children in Primary and Secondary Care*, London, Royal College of General Practitioners.

The National Society for Epilepsy, available online at *www.epilepsynse.org.uk/pages/info/leaflets/epfacts.cfm*.

Wood, T. (1994) 'Weight Status of a Group of Adults with Learning Disabilities', *British Journal of Learning Disabilities*, **22**: 97–9.

7 Health Promotion Perspectives for Adults with Learning Disabilities

DEBRA FEARNS, JACKIE KELLY, PAUL MALORET, MALCOLM McIVER AND TRACEY-JO SIMPSON

KEY POINTS

- There is clear evidence that many healthcare needs of adults with learning disabilities remain unmet.
- There is low reporting of illnesses and symptoms among adults with learning disabilities, with the subsequent risk of misdiagnosis and inappropriate treatment, or no treatment at all.
- A key aspect of the role of those who care for and support adults with learning disabilities is to convey health promotion messages at an appropriate level that the service user can understand.
- Women who have learning disabilities are less likely to undergo cervical smear tests than the general population.

INTRODUCTION

It is known that adults with learning disabilities are more likely to have greater additional physical needs than the general population. For example, as outlined in Chapter 8, we know that adults with Down's syndrome are at an increased risk of recurrent chest infections, congenital heart defects and anaemia. Epilepsy is also present in one-third of adults with learning disabilities, yet only 0.5 per cent of the general population have epilepsy (Department of Health 2001a). Adults with learning disabilities are also living to an older age, and hence developing associated age-related health needs.

Yet, there is clear evidence that many healthcare needs of adults with learning disabilities remain unmet, as highlighted by the National Health Service Executive (NHSE) paper, *Signposts for Success* and most recently in the government's White Paper, *Valuing People* (Department of Health 2001a).

These unmet needs may be due to a number of factors, and include:

Caring for People with Learning Disabilities. Edited by I. Peate and D. Fearns.
Copyright © 2006 by John Wiley & Sons, Ltd.

- communication difficulties;
- inability of carers to recognise the health needs of adults with learning disabilities;
- general practitioners (GPs) not understanding fully the healthcare needs of their patients who have learning disabilities;
- general ignorance about the specific healthcare needs of adults with learning disabilities;
- prejudice from carers and professionals towards adults with learning disabilities.

BARRIERS TO ACCESSING HEALTH CARE

In spite of recent legislation and advances in the provision of care, the evidence suggests that the healthcare needs of adults with learning disabilities are still not being fully met:

- Adults with learning disabilities are much more likely to be obese than the general population.
- Less than 10 per cent of adults with learning disabilities eat a balanced diet, with an insufficient intake of fruit and vegetables and a lack of knowledge and choice about healthy eating.
- Less than 20 per cent of adults with learning disabilities engage in physical activity at or above the minimum level recommended by the Department of Health, as opposed to 36 per cent of the general population (Robertson et al. 2000).

> '70% of people with learning disabilities visit their GP four or less times a year. The average for the general population is five times a year'.
>
> (Band 1998)

Adults with learning disabilities are less likely to receive regular health checks (Whitfield et al. 1996), and are 58 times more likely to die before the age of 50 years than those without a learning disability, often from preventable conditions such as respiratory illness (Hollins et al. 1998). It is little wonder that the Disability Rights Commission felt moved to say:

> '... there is compelling evidence of inequalities in health outcomes between disabled and non-disabled people; and evidence of significant problems in access, staff attitudes and quality of service.'
>
> (Disability Rights Commission 2004)

That adults with learning disabilities die younger than non-disabled people is an established fact, yet learning disability in itself is not a cause of premature death. Adults with learning disabilities are more likely to die young because of deprivation, lifestyle and *barriers to accessing health promotion, assessment, screening and treatment*. For example, whilst 77 per cent of women in the general population routinely undergo cervical smears, for women with a learning disability, that figure is only 19 per cent (Djuretic et al. 1999). Similarly, they are much less likely to engage in breast cancer examinations, and receive far fewer (33 per cent) invites to mammography than women without a learning disability (Davies & Duff 2001).

So what are the barriers that prevent adults with learning disabilities accessing the health services that they need? Ironically, the answer appears to be the very professionals who are supposed to be helping them.

Despite the fact that 75 per cent of GPs have had no training in treating adults with learning disabilities, 90 per cent of them believe that a learning disability makes diagnosis harder. Mencap (2004) report that many families of people with learning disabilities state that some doctors look at their son or daughter and – consciously or unconsciously – believe that his/her health problem is a result of the learning disability and that not much can be done about it. As a consequence, there is a low reporting of illnesses and symptoms among adults with learning disabilities, with the subsequent risk of misdiagnosis and inappropriate treatment, or no treatment at all (Beange et al. 1999).

A lack of accessible information further adds to the barriers that adults with learning disabilities face. Despite the fact that all but the smallest of GP practices are likely to have upwards of 40 patients with learning disabilities (NHSE 1999), 70 per cent do not provide any accessible information (Mencap 2004). With little understanding of their needs and no access to understandable information, it is not surprising that 20 per cent of disabled people find it difficult or impossible to access health care. One in seven could not collect prescriptions and 20 per cent had deferred treatment, compared with just 7 per cent of the general population (Leonard Cheshire 2003).

Some adults with learning disabilities lead unhealthy lifestyles which hinder attempts to live a healthy life. This can be partly explained by the fact that many adults with learning disabilities rely on carers and family members to shop, cook and provide meals and to help them undertake activities. Often, this results in adults with learning disabilities leading a sedentary lifestyle (Mencap 2004). Despite government initiatives, adults with learning disabilities are poorly served by primary and secondary healthcare provision. There has been a tendency for specialist NHS services to develop their own inclusive services. However, this model of provision continues to segregate adults with learning disabilities from mainstream services and has 'allowed' the NHS to continue to ignore their needs (Department of Health 2001a).

ATTITUDINAL BARRIERS

Adults with learning disabilities are a marginalised group within society, and, unfortunately, this is reflected in attitudes expressed by professional health and social care staff. Shanley and Guest (1995) highlighted that adults with learning disabilities are stigmatised by adult nurses. Slevin and Sines (1996) reported that adult nurses showed an unenthusiastic attitude towards people with learning disabilities. This may be explained, in part, by their lack of exposure to adults with learning disabilities and that even in a 'Common Foundation Programme' (CFP), the majority of content and teaching centred on adult nurses. It is possible, though, that even with a more balanced CFP and exposure to adults with learning disabilities in a short practice experience, these attitudes may still not change. Fitzsimmons and Barr (1997) identified a number of factors that could influence attitudes. These included: poor preparation and education and awareness of people with learning disabilities; communication barriers; difficulties in dealing with their behaviour; and limited understanding of what constitutes learning disabilities.

Other health and social care professionals may also have stigmatising attitudes towards adults with learning disabilities which need to be challenged. This is evidenced by the report *Facing the Facts* (Department of Health 1999), which details that health professionals were 'not in tune with the way that people with learning disabilities experience health interventions'. It is hoped that the strategies outlined by the Department of Health (2001a) will help to foster effective working relationships that will promote understanding and overcome stigmatisation. Later sections in this chapter will highlight good practice initiatives that are being put in place to support adults with learning disabilities.

HEALTH PROMOTION APPROACHES

'Health promotion refers to a group of activities that help to prevent disease and improve health and well being' (Naidoo & Wills 2000). Elements of health promotion centre on disease prevention, health education and health information, public health promotion and community development. However, there are barriers to health promotion that need to be understood and challenged. From the service users' perspective, these may include:

- lack of knowledge or understanding and communication skills
- inappropriate and inaccessible services
- physical disabilities.

From the professionals' perspective, these may include:

- lack of knowledge and poor communication skills
- restrictions on their time
- set ways of working.

(Shaughnessy & Cruse 2001)

Within these perspectives, it is important to note that the adult with a learning disability has the right to expect the same level of service as an adult in the general population receives, regardless of barriers that may be in place. The King's Fund (1980) has argued that adults with learning disabilities have equal value to any other individual and this is reinforced by the White Paper *Valuing People* (Department of Health 2001a).

Health promotion aims to improve health and manage or prevent disease, using a deliberate approach (Tones & Tilford 1994). Health promotion is often targeted at specific health issues, aimed at the general public. The government commonly sets targets, such as reducing the number of teenage pregnancies or reducing deaths from coronary heart disease. Adults with learning disabilities may coincidentally be involved, but they are not specifically targeted. This becomes problematic when primary care staff and services fail to adopt strategies to include adults with learning disabilities. Shaughnessy and Cruse (2001) note that there needs to be a major shift in attitude from professional staff, carers and service users. They also point out that improvements for adults with learning disabilities will be improved by effective inter-agency teamwork, centred on the needs of adults with learning disabilities.

As carers and students, an essential role when working with adults with learning disabilities is to ensure that they have access to all health provision, as and when required. Indeed, it is a fundamental right, and is crucial in ensuring that adults with learning disabilities are participating and included as members of our community (O'Brien 1987). There are challenges ahead, but learning disability nurses need to demonstrate to those whom they support and care for that their role is critical in guaranteeing appropriate and timely interventions that sustain healthy lifestyles and access high-quality health care when ill, ultimately leading to the optimal health status for that individual.

A key aspect of the role of those who care for and support adults with learning disability is to convey health promotion messages at an appropriate level that the service user can understand. It may be commonly understood by the general public that eating five portions of fruit and vegetables per day is desirable as part of a balanced diet. Explaining this concept to a service user who is used to chips and beans requires the carer to deliver the message appropriately and sensibly. If the service user has a limited budget, telling him/her to change his/her eating habits will not result in a change in behaviour. Going shopping with him/her, devising menus and targeting specific changes that the service user can experience as making a difference will be much more effective in helping to modify lifestyle. These methods are supportive of 'positive and healthy lifestyles' (Cowley 1996), health promotion activities that stress the importance of self-determination and encourage independence and choice.

HEALTH SCREENING FOR PEOPLE WHO HAVE LEARNING DISABILITIES

Since the late 1980s, there have been numerous reports highlighting unmet health needs for people who have learning disabilities (Howells 1986). There is also evidence of the poor uptake of screening services nationally (Whitfield et al. 1996). Women who have learning disabilities are less likely to undergo cervical smear tests than the general population – 19 compared with 77 per cent (Djuretic et al. 1999) – and, despite a 90 per cent attendance rate at mammography clinics, are less likely to engage in breast examinations or receive invitations to mammography than the general population (Davies & Duff 2001). Many stereotypical reasons exist to back the theory, such as the assumption that:

- the women are not engaging in sexual intercourse;
- the tests would be too distressing;
- the person would not understand what was happening.

Unfortunately, the above remarks are too often given when care workers, nurses and relatives ask for the reasons why the person whom they support and care for is not given the same screening rights as any other person in the United Kingdom.

To date, there is no screening test for testicular cancer but men above the age of 18 years should be encouraged to self-examine, although with figures of between 3 per cent in family care and 6 per cent in formal care settings who have undertaken testicular examinations, it probably highlights the difficulties that carers have about such an intimate procedure.

Health Minister Rosie Winterton announced that from April 2006, a national bowel cancer screening programme would be phased in. Men and women aged 60–69 years will be screened every two years. With an ageing population in learning disabilities, it is also vital that people are accessing this screening programme in the months to come.

Many individuals who have learning disabilities attend their GP surgeries less often than the general population, with many individuals relying on others to observe changes in their health or behaviours and make appointments accordingly. Many surgeries are often unaware of any additional support needs that individuals may have in order to read the invitations, discuss what the screening is for and understand personal responsibilities for health care, with the onus being placed on carers to provide such information. This often results in many people not attending appointments compared with the general population.

Since the publication of *Valuing People* (Department of Health 2001a), many primary healthcare and specialist trusts have introduced named health facilitators to meet the government's objective of enabling mainstream services to meet the general and specialist health needs of people who have learning disabilities. Health facilitation and Health Action Plans (HAPs) (Department of Health 2002a, 2002b) are just two initiatives that could improve the care of people who have learning disabilities in mainstream settings. This will be discussed in more detail in a later section. Other local initiatives include learning disability nurses placed within general hospitals to provide the localised support for both the individual and the medical team from admission to discharge. Learning disability nurses completing health visitor qualifications are being placed with strategic health promotion roles within health authorities.

All of these initiatives require extra funding; the government announced in February 2005 that it would be providing £41 million for primary care trusts to develop their services for people who have learning disabilities. Stephen Ladyman said:

'I am very pleased to announce that funding for the Learning Disabilities Development Fund has almost doubled for the coming year. These funds are intended to support the implementation of the Government white paper "Valuing People", which sets out a wide ranging programme of action to improve services for people with learning disabilities based on four key principles – rights, independence, choice and inclusion.'

Part of that inclusion is for individuals to understand their rights to healthcare provision such as health screening. Many women who have learning disabilities attend screening tests and do not understand the purpose of the test (Broughton & Thomson 2000). Surely, personal inclusion in healthcare has to consider informed consent with regard to any procedures being carried out. The Department of Health has issued a number of guidance documents to assist in the process of seeking consent from people who have learning disabilities (Department of Health 2001b). Unfortunately, people's reluctance to engage in the screening process is often interpreted as a personal choice or refusal and therefore no further support is given to the individual. With the advent of the Mental Capacity Act 2005, coming into force in 2007, the Act introduces a 'new criminal offence of ill treatment or neglect of a person who lacks capacity. A person found guilty of such an offence may be liable to imprisonment for a term of up to five years'. This may 'force' services to reconsider their interpretation of someone's reluctance and find more appropriate ways of providing information to individuals, such as picture booklets (NHS Cancer Screening Programmes 2000a, 2000b), videos, role-play sessions and de-sensitisation sessions.

Many people can make informed choices given the right support and information but this takes time and effort from all sides. Health screening requires us all to provide that time and effort if people who have learning disabilities are to be afforded the same rights to health care as the general population.

HEALTH FACILITATION

Valuing People (Department of Health 2001a) clearly states the existence of inequalities in health and in healthcare delivery for adults with learning disabilities. It sets out guidance that incorporates key principles of rights, independence, choice and inclusion for adults with learning disabilities. The emphasis is very much on social inclusion, and this extends to the areas of health care and healthcare delivery. Adults with learning disabilities should expect to have the same support in relation to their health needs as anyone else. Historically, the health experience and life expectancy of people with these additional complications were potentially poor. However, improvements in health care have meant that people can now expect to live longer with appropriate healthcare intervention, and hence the need to ensure that equal access to such health care is facilitated for adults who have learning disabilities.

To achieve this, an inter-agency approach is proposed and adopted. Partnership Boards were established within each local authority area, consisting of public, private, community and voluntary sector representatives, with a clear remit to involve adults with learning disabilities and their carers in the planning and implementation of the health agenda for adults with learning disabilities within their areas.

Through Partnership Boards, the implementation of the Health Action Plan process began and continues to address the issues of healthcare needs for adults with learning disabilities.

Health Action Plans are individual plans adopted within the concept of a person-centred approach to care. Health Action Plans identify the health needs of an individual and clearly indicate the support necessary to address those needs and optimise the health experience of the individual.

The person who has a learning disability, with a health facilitator(s), develops these plans. Health facilitators are identified within each Primary Care Trust; these individuals work as a bridge between the adult with a learning disability, mainstream healthcare services and specialist learning disability services, as appropriate. Their role is to ensure that each person has a Health Action Plan, and subsequently the opportunity to access appropriate healthcare support.

As noted above, the emphasis within accessing health care is based within the principle of inclusion. Where possible, adults with learning disabilities are *facilitated* to utilise mainstream health services, such as local GP services, rather than feeling segregated within 'specialist' services. It is hard to believe that not all adults with learning disabilities have been registered with a GP in the past. This fact in itself highlights the inequality that people have historically experienced. Indeed, the Department of Health's *Good Practice Guidance* (2002b), relating to Health Action Plans and health facilitation, clearly states that there has been a reluctance in some mainstream healthcare services to support improving health for adults with learning disabilities. This reluctance can often relate to concerns about lack of time, skills or adequate resources. However, this resistance is now being addressed through the work of health facilitators, providing information, education and support to enable greater identification of the health needs of adults with learning disabilities within our community.

Who might these health facilitators be? Within the White Paper (Department of Health 2001a), the community learning disability nurse (CLDN) is identified as a key professional who may be well placed (though not exclusively) to take on the health facilitation role. The CLDN often works within a multidisciplinary context in a community-based team, with access to the advice and support of a variety of professionals, such as consultant psychiatrists, clinical psychologists, speech and language therapists, occupational therapists, social workers and counsellors. They have a broad knowledge base in respect of the potential health needs of adults with learning disabilities. They may have established networks liaising in an inter-professional capacity with the primary healthcare team, for example. The facilitation of optimum health for the adults with whom they work will already form part of their portfolio of expertise.

A key role for the health facilitator is close working with local GPs, enabling them to identify the healthcare needs of the people with learning disabilities registered within their practice. Ensuring that people with learning disabilities have access to GP care and enabling people with learning disabilities to complete Health Action Plans and be involved in the decisions made in respect of their health care is also part of their role.

It is important to note the issue of inclusion here once again. Though every effort should be made to facilitate the individual to access mainstream services, *Valuing People* (Department of Health 2001a) also notes that there are times when specialist services may be better placed in terms of knowledge, skills, experience or appropriateness of care to support adults with particular aspects of their healthcare needs. As carers or students supporting people with learning disabilities, you need to be conscious that a person's experience of health and healthcare provision is an individual one. In your work with adults with learning disabilities, you will need to be aware of the local health facilitators and related resources, to enable people to access appropriate support. Facilitating the achievement of optimum health should be everyone's aim. Including the person in his/her Health Action Plan, and ensuring that the most appropriate service provides that care, be that specialist or mainstream services, will enable this to happen.

HEALTH IMPROVEMENT CLINICS

Healthcare professionals working with adults with learning disabilities have been increasingly concerned with their interface with primary and secondary health care over the last decade. Notably, the 'Survey of GPs' Views of Learning Disability Services' (Marshal et al. 1996) highlights the disappointing attitudes of GPs toward adults with learning disabilities who attempt to access a service from the Primary Care Trust. *Our Healthier Nation* (Department of Health 1998) acknowledges that adults with learning disabilities are a 'vulnerable group' and set out to make vast improvements before 2010. Since the time of these publications, much has been written about the problem and, consequently, many initiatives within services for adults with learning disabilities have been undertaken, with varying degrees of success. One initiative that has certainly had a positive impact for adults with learning disabilities is the 'Health Improvement Clinic'.

The clinic provides an opportunity for those who experience access problems for a variety of reasons to receive a comprehensive health assessment and, if required, an action plan aimed at meeting their highlighted health needs. It is important to note that the intention of these clinics is not to replace primary care or secondary care services for adults with learning disabilities, but instead to support them. *Valuing People* (Department of Health 2001a) identifies primary care services as the first point of contact for adults with learning disabilities.

However, Gates (2003) identifies a variety of issues from a service user's perspective which may act as 'barriers' to receiving a good service from a GP surgery. Many of these are based on the 'fear' or 'anxieties' which exist amongst many adults with learning disabilities. These include being fearful of the environment of the GP surgery, which has been described as a very 'serious' and 'unwelcoming place', and, also, the doctors themselves may appear quite authoritarian and very often are a complete stranger to their learning disabled patients. Additionally, difficulties occur with communication, as, often, the GP is extremely time-constricted and cannot take the time to learn to understand the patient and too often communicates via an accompanying carer to save time, which can leave the patient feeling undermined.

It is for these reasons that the Health Improvement Clinic will usually take place in a location which is familiar to the user, such as day centres, colleges, places of work and their homes. The clinic is usually led by two learning disability nurses, who are usually familiar with the location and the users within it. However, it is not unusual to see the same people on a number of occasions within the clinic to help them get used to the idea of the clinic and the nurses. The clinic utilises a referral system whereby service users are encouraged to self-refer and highlight areas of health need which may require closer attention. For each referral, an appointment lasting approximately an hour is allocated. It was found that this was a reasonable time span in which to complete a thorough health check. Generally speaking, the 'OK' Health Check (Matthews 2004) or similarities are utilised. Matthews and Hegarty (1997) explain that the 'OK' Health Check is designed to systematically assess areas of health in which adults with learning disabilities are particularly vulnerable; they are listed in Table 7.1.

Routinely, it is usual for the nurses to check temperature, pulse and respirations. Urine is tested, as are the glucose levels in the blood. Additionally, some clinics offer a phlebotomy service; this normally depends upon the nature of the referral or the assessment findings.

Because of the 'sexuality issues' discussed in this assessment, it is advisable, where possible, for a male nurse to work alongside a female nurse. Following the assessment, the nurses will discuss the results and the appropriate action plan with the service user and his/her carer, if this is deemed appropriate. It is important to note that the information gathered is confidential and it should never be assumed that anyone else in attendance at the clinic should be informed of the results or the action plan. In all instances, consent is sought to communicate the results to the service user's GP. The principal purpose of this is to allow for any GP opinion on the results and action plan, thus improving partnership working between the primary care teams and the

Table 7.1. The areas of health assessed by the 'OK' Health Check (source: Matthews 1998)

- Current medication and side effects
- Circulation and breathing
- Perception of pain
- Digestion and elimination
- Skin condition
- Feet
- Ears and hearing
- Sexuality issues
- Lifestyle risks
- Body dimension and measurement
- Epilepsy
- Urinary system
- Physique and mobility
- Oral hygiene
- Eyes and vision
- Mental health
- Sleep

learning disability services. McKenzie and Powell (2004) emphasise the need for primary care teams to work with learning disability teams to provide good quality health care for adults with learning disabilities.

The action plan is often diverse in nature and could be a referral to an appropriate agency or professional. This referral may be internal, i.e. to another member of the learning disability team, such as a psychiatrist or therapist. Alternatively, it may be an external referral perhaps to a member of the primary care team, such as a chiropodist or a dentist, as appropriate. In all instances, the nurses would allow for time to discuss the most suitable way to support the referred agency and the service user, as, often, support and a certain amount of creativity are required, enhancing the chances of success. For some, using the clinic is a desensitisation process to eventually utilising GP surgeries and therefore may need to return to the clinic in a GP surgery. The information recorded can also be transferred on the service user's Health Action Plan – another initiative discussed within this chapter.

Additionally, the clinic acts as an advisory service on health issues and aims to promote health. Powrie (2003) highlights the need for health promotional information in general to be more 'user friendly towards adults with learning disability', stating that a recent analysis of leaflets held in GP surgeries showed there was very little that could be described as educationally informing to those with difficulties in reading and understanding. The learning disability nurses are in constant liaison with health promotional agencies that provide 'user-friendly' material; this is made available at the clinics.

NATIONAL PATIENT SAFETY AGENCY

The National Patient Safety Agency (NPSA) has, in recent times, published its report outlining key patient safety issues in relation to the quality of care of adults with learning disabilities in a number of areas, including physical restraint (NPSA 2004). The focus of this section concerns the 'vulnerability of people with learning disabilities in general hospitals'. One of the problems it highlights concerns the 'degree of harm' that adults with learning disabilities may come across as patients in a general hospital. It reports that 26 per cent of adults with learning disabilities are admitted to hospital every year. This compares with 14 per cent in the general population (Band 1998). The NPSA states that a number of concerns were raised, including:

- communication difficulties;
- inadequate training in specific health concerns;
- additional health conditions, such as epilepsy and not being recognised in general hospitals;

- reliance on carers and learning disability professionals to carry out full nursing care;
- consent being sought from the carer, and not the persons themselves.

(NPSA 2004)

These are worrying issues and, coupled with a lack of accessible information and illnesses either misdiagnosed or undiagnosed, highlight the work that still needs to be done to improve how health professionals interact with adults with learning disabilities. The NPSA can voice its concerns at a national level and promote the issues affecting adults with learning disabilities in accessing secondary care.

CONCLUSION

Adults with learning disabilities have more unmet healthcare needs than the general population, yet face barriers in accessing primary and secondary health services. Despite recent government reports and initiatives, much remains to be done to improve access to services. These include challenging physical barriers as well as attitudinal barriers. *Valuing People* (Department of Health 2001a) sets out key points that need improvement, but inclusion in health screening and surveillance, health promotion and access to generic services remain a challenge. As carers and students, we need to work cooperatively with professionals and organisations to increase knowledge and awareness of the health needs of adults with learning disabilities and how these can be best addressed. Health facilitators and Patients Advice and Liaison Services (PALS) can help make a difference. However, real change will come from learning disability nurses, students and carers advocating for change and educating health professionals in understanding the needs of people with learning disabilities.

REFERENCES

Band, R. (1998) *The NHS: Health for All?*, research report, London, Mencap.

Beange, H., Lennox, N. & Parmenter, T. (1999) 'Health Targets for People with an Intellectual Disability', *Journal of Intellectual and Developmental Disability*, **24**(4): 283–98.

Broughton, S. & Thomson, K. (2000) 'Women with Learning Disabilities: Risk Behaviours and Experiences of the Cervical Smear Test', *Journal of Advanced Nursing*, **32**: 905–12.

Cowley, S. (1996) 'Promoting Positive and Healthy Lifestyles', in S. Twinn, B. Roberts & S. Andrews (eds), *Community Health Care Nursing: Principles for Practice*, London, Butterworth Heinemann, Chapter 26.

Davies, N. & Duff, M. (2001) 'Breast Cancer Screening for Older Women with Intellectual Disability Living in Community Group Homes', *Journal of Intellectual Disability Research*, **45**(3): 253–7.

Department of Health (1998) *Our Healthier Nation*, London, The Stationery Office.

Department of Health (1999) *Facing the Facts*, London, Department of Health.

Department of Health (2001a) *Valuing People: A New Strategy for Learning Disability for the 21st Century*, London, The Stationery Office.

Department of Health (2001b) *Seeking Consent: Working with People with Learning Disabilities*, London, The Stationery Office.

Department of Health (2002a) *Action for Health: Health Action Plans and Health Facilitation – Detailed Good Practice Guidance on Implementation for Learning Disability Partnership Boards*, London, HMSO.

Department of Health (2002b) *Health Action Plans and Health Facilitation: Good Practice Guidance for Learning Disability Partnership Boards – Easier to Read Version*, London, HMSO.

Disability Rights Commission (2004) *Discriminating Treatment? Disabled People and the Health Service*, Disability Rights Commission.

Djuretic, T., Laing-Mroto, T. & Guy, M. (1999) 'Concerted Effort is Needed to Ensure these Women Use Preventive Services' [letter], *British Medical Journal*, **318**: 536.

Fitzsimmons, J. & Barr, O. (1997) 'A Review of the Reported Attitudes of Health and Social Care Professionals towards People with Learning Disabilities: Implications for Education and Further Research', *Journal of Learning Disabilities for Nursing, Health and Social Care*, **1**(2): 57–64.

Gates, B. (2003) *Learning Disabilities: Towards Inclusion*, London, Churchill Livingstone.

Grant, G., Goward, P., Richardson, M. & Ramcharan, P. (2005) *Learning Disability A Life Cycle Approach to Valuing People*, London, Oxford University Press.

Hollins, S., Attard, M. T., von Fraunhofer, N., McGuigan, S. & Sedgwick, P. (1998) 'Mortality in People with Learning Disability: Risks, Causes, and Death Certification Findings in London', *Developmental Medicine and Child Neurology*, **40**(1): 50–6.

Howells, G. (1986) 'Are the Medical Needs of Mentally Handicapped Adults Being Met?', *Journal of the Royal College of General Practitioners*, **36**: 449–53.

King's Fund (1980) *An Ordinary Life: Comprehensive Locally-Based Services for Mentally Handicapped People*, London, King's Fund.

Leonard Cheshire (2003) *Mind the Gap: The Leonard Cheshire Social Exclusion Report 2003*, Leonard Cheshire.

Marshal, S., Martin, D. & Myles, F. (1996) 'Survey of GPs' Views of Learning Disability Services', *British Journal of Nursing*, **5**(13): 798–800, 802–4.

Matthews, D. R. (2004) *'OK' Health Check: Health Facilitation and Health Action Planning*, 3rd edn, Preston, Fairfield.

Matthews, D. & Hegarty, J. (1997) ' "OK" Health Check: Health Assessment Checklist for People with Learning Disabilities', *British Journal of Learning Disabilities*, **25**(4): 138–43.

McKenzie, K. & Powell, H. (2004) 'Screen Health', *Learning Disability Practice*, **7**(10).

Mencap (2004) *Treat Me Right! Better Healthcare for People with a Learning Disability*, Mencap.

Naidoo, J. & Wills, J. (2000) *Health Promotion: Foundations for Practice*, 2nd edn, London, Bailliere Tindall.

NHS Cancer Screening Programmes (2000a) *50 or Over? Breast Screening is for You*, NHS.

NHS Cancer Screening Programmes (2000b) *Having a Smear Test*, NHS.

NHS Executive (1999) *Once a Day: One or More People with Learning Disabilities Are Likely to Be in Contact with your Primary Healthcare Team: How Can You Help Them?*, London, Department of Health.

NPSA (National Patient Safety Agency) (2004) *Listening to People with Learning Difficulties and Family Carers Talk about Patient Safety*, London, NPSA.

O'Brien, J. (1987) 'A Guide to Personal Futures Planning', in G. T. Bellamy & B. Wilcox (eds), *The Activities Catalogue*, Georgia, USA, Responsive Systems Associates.

Powrie, E. (2003) 'Primary Health Care Provision for Adults with Learning Disability', *Journal of Advanced Nursing*, **42**(4): 413–23.

Robertson, J., Emerson, E., Gregory, N., Hatton, C., Turner, S., Kessissoglou, S. & Hallam, A. (2000) 'Lifestyle Related Risk Factors for Poor Health in Residential Settings for People with Intellectual Disabilities', *Research in Developmental Disabilities*, **21**: 469–86.

Shanley, E. & Guest, C. (1995) 'Stigmatisation of People with Learning Disabilities in General Hospitals', *British Journal of Nursing*, **13**: 759–60.

Shaughnessy, P. & Cruse, S. (2001) 'Health Promotion with People Who Have a Learning Disability', in J. Thompson & S. Pickering (eds), *Meeting the Health Needs of People Who Have a Learning Disability*, London, Bailliere Tindall, pp. 126–57.

Slevin, E. & Sines, D. (1996) 'Attitudes of Nurses in a General Hospital towards People with Learning Disabilities', *Journal of Advanced Nursing*, **24**: 1116–26.

Tones, K. & Tilford, S. (1994) *Health Education, Effectiveness, Efficiency and Equity*, London, Chapman and Hall.

Whitfield, M., Langan, J. & Russell, O. (1996) 'Assessing GPs' Care of Adult Patients with a Learning Disability: Case-Control Study', *Quality in Health Care*, **5**(1): 31–5.

8 The Biophysical Aspects of Learning Disabilities

FRANK GARVEY AND JACKY VINCENT

KEY POINTS

- Adults with learning disabilities have greater health needs than non-learning disabled adults and are prone to chronic health problems.
- Adults with learning disabilities are 58 times more likely to die before the age of 50 years than are non-learning disabled adults.
- Effective communication and information sharing are central to the effective meeting of health needs of adults with learning disabilities.
- In some instances, treatable diseases may go undetected, progressing until the treatment required is less effective.
- Down's syndrome offers a model of approach that can be transferred to other adults with learning disabilities.

INTRODUCTION

The learning disability strategic document the White Paper *Valuing People* (Department of Health 2001) and the report *Treat Me Right* (Mencap 2004) are amongst many recent papers highlighting the fact that adults with learning disabilities have greater health needs than non-learning disabled adults and are prone to chronic health problems, epilepsy and physical and sensory disabilities. Although adults with learning disabilities have a similar range of healthcare conditions to non-learning disabled adults, they are two-and-a-half times more likely to have a condition – often of a higher prevalence (Kerr 1998; Martin et al. 1997), requiring medical attention (Van Schrojenstein et al. 2000). Table 8.1 outlines the most significant secondary conditions.

Hollins et al. (1998) state that adults with learning disabilities are 58 times more likely to die before the age of 50 years than are non-learning disabled adults. One of the reasons for this is that treatable diseases remain undetected until they have progressed to a stage at which the treatment required is less effective. In addition, adults with learning disabilities access their general practitioner (GP) far less frequently than the general population, even though their health needs are greater. Even when visiting GPs, barriers to effective

Caring for People with Learning Disabilities. Edited by I. Peate and D. Fearns.
Copyright © 2006 by John Wiley & Sons, Ltd.

Table 8.1. Twenty most significant secondary
conditions (source: Frey et al. 2001)

- Communication difficulties
- Persistence problems
- Weight problems
- Personal hygiene/appearance
- Physical fitness and conditioning
- Fatigue
- Dental hygiene
- Sleep problems and disturbances
- Balance problems/dizziness
- Joint and muscle pain
- Contractures
- Bowel dysfunction
- Bladder dysfunction
- Depression
- Mobility problems
- Memory problems
- Injuries due to accidents and/or seizures
- Injuries due to self-harm
- Vision problems
- Medication side effects

treatment can occur, such as communication difficulties, pressures on time and GPs' not appreciating the additional health conditions that co-exist for many adults with learning disabilities, leading to a missed or incorrect diagnosis.

This chapter provides an overview of the 'biophysical aspects' of learning disability, with a particular focus upon the physical health issues of adults with Down's syndrome. It is intended that the reader will be then be able to draw inferences across a range of learning disability syndromes. 'Medical' terms are used alongside 'physical' descriptions and it is hoped that further reading using these terms will occur.

Where a learning disability is caused (the aetiology) by a genetic or chromosomal abnormality, disease and illness (pathology) are usually present. Pathologies can affect both the structure (anatomy) and the function (physiology) of a variety of bodily systems. As carers, students and professionals, using knowledge of the human body and its associated pathologies can support preventative, efficient and effective healthcare, ensuring that it is provided in an equitable way.

Down's syndrome is a relatively common chromosomal condition that, in addition to causing learning disability, results in a high number of associated physical health conditions (co-morbidity) across the lifespan. The ageing process is known to be hastened, with adults with Down's syndrome being physiologically 10–20 years in advance of their chronological age. Furthermore, adults with Down's syndrome are more prone to autoimmune diseases, such as diabetes mellitus, hypothyroidism and coeliac disease, as well as musculoskeletal, skin and heart disorders. It is important that these factors are considered when caring for adults with Down's syndrome, as they may impact on their health and well-being throughout their lifespan. Understanding these particular conditions will maximise optimal health and well-being for adults with Down's syndrome, ensuring a better representation of their needs when interfacing with primary and secondary care providers.

MUSCULOSKELETAL DISORDERS

Almost all of the conditions that affect the bones and joints of adults with Down's syndrome arise from the abnormal collagen found in adults with Down's syndrome. Collagen is the major protein that makes up ligaments, tendons, cartilage, bone and the support structure of the skin. One type of collagen (type VI) is encoded by a gene found on the 21st chromosome. The effect in adults with Down's syndrome is increased laxity, or looseness, of the ligaments that attach bone to bone and muscle to bone. The combination of this ligamentous laxity and low muscle tone contribute to orthopaedic problems in adults with Down's syndrome. While these conditions are more common in adults with Down's syndrome than in the general population, the majority of adults with Down's syndrome will not have any of these disorders.

SPINE

The major condition associated with the spine in Down's syndrome is atlantoaxial instability, which is the looseness between the first and second vertebrae of the neck.

Atlantoaxial instability (AAI) in Down's syndrome

AAI denotes increased mobility at the articulation of the first and second cervical vertebrae (atlantoaxial joint). The causes of AAI are not well understood but may include abnormalities of the ligaments that maintain the integrity of the articulation, bony abnormalities of the cervical vertebrae, or both.

In its mildest form, AAI is asymptomatic and is diagnosed using x-rays. Symptomatic AAI results from subluxation (excessive slippage that is severe enough to injure the spinal cord) or from dislocation at the atlantoaxial joint.

Approximately 15 per cent of youths with Down's syndrome have AAI. Almost all are asymptomatic. The neurological manifestations of atlantoaxial instability include tiredness, difficulty in walking, abnormal gait, neck pain, limited neck mobility and head tilting to one side (torticollis), poor coordination, clumsiness, and sensory deficits. Nearly all of the individuals who have experienced serious injury to the spinal cord have had a long history reflecting the above outlined clinical picture. There is no evidence that participating in sporting activities increases the risk of cervical spine injuries (Department of Health 1995). In the event of an individual's requiring general anaesthesia, nursing and medical staff should be alerted to the possibility of atlantoaxial instability so as to provide the necessary support when moving and handling the unconscious patient (Casey et al. 1995). In a few instances, this may be severe enough to traumatise the spinal cord, with resultant sensory and motor neuronal damage (Davidson 1988), loss of control of bowel or bladder, and spasticity.

Most importantly, symptomatic AAI is apparently rare in individuals with Down's syndrome. Carers and students must learn the symptoms of AAI, outlined above, that indicate the need to seek immediate medical care.

Scoliosis

This is another condition associated with the spine in adults with Down's syndrome. It means curvature of the spine to the side. While it appears to be more common in adults with Down's syndrome, the exact incidence isn't known. In the era when almost all children with Down's syndrome were institutionalised, scoliosis may have been seen in up to half of them as they became adolescents. Bracing is the initial treatment of scoliosis but if necessary, as determined by the orthopaedic surgeon, this can be followed by surgical intervention.

HIP

Legg–Calve–Perthes (LCP) is a disorder of the hip, in which the head of the femur loses its blood supply and the bone becomes weak and misshapen. LCP is slightly more common in children with Down's syndrome than in the general population. This condition usually presents as a painless limp and loss of full range of movement of the involved hip. It is diagnosed through x-rays. Mild cases or cases discovered early may be treated with a combination of bed rest, orthotics and casting. Severe cases require surgical correction.

Slipped capital femoral epiphysis (SCFE, also called epiphysiolysis) can be seen in adults with Down's syndrome less frequently. In this condition, the rounded head of the femur slides on the neck of the femur. This condition can be associated with obesity and hypothyroidism, both of which are common in teenagers and adults with Down's syndrome. SCFE appears as a limp with associated pain in the hip or knee (hip conditions often cause knee pain instead of hip pain), and is treated by surgical replacement of the femur.

KNEE

Instability of the patella (kneecap) has been estimated to occur in almost 20 per cent of adults with Down's syndrome. The majority of cases of instability present only as kneecaps that can be moved further to the outside than the normal kneecap (subluxation); however, some adults can have their kneecaps completely moved out of position (dislocation) and some may even have a hard time getting them back into the right position. Mild subluxation of the kneecap is not associated with pain, but dislocation may be painful. While adults with instability of the patella are able to walk, there is often a decreased range of motion of the knee, with an accompanying change in gait. The longer that nothing is done for the instability, the worse the condition will get over time. Orthoses (special braces) may be useful for mild cases, but severe cases require surgical correction.

FEET

Flat foot (pes planus) is seen in the vast majority of adults with Down's syndrome. In mild cases, the heel is in a neutral position. In severe cases, the heel rotates so that the person is walking on the inside of the heel. Flat feet result in heavy calluses of the feet, pointing of the front part of the feet away from each other (the opposite of being 'pigeon-toed'), and even the creation of bone spurs in the feet. Many cases respond to orthotics, but severe cases need surgical correction.

Metatarsus primus varus (MPV) is also commonly seen in adults with Down's syndrome, and is the condition in which the front part of the foot behind the big toe bends inward. This creates an obvious deformity of the foot, making the task of finding shoes that fit more difficult. If the condition exists for long enough, a painful irritation called a bunion appears at the spot where the foot bends in the most. Mild or early cases of MPV may be treated with orthotics or special shoes, but severe cases require surgical correction.

In these situations, it is important to ensure that adults with Down's syndrome have properly fitting shoes that do not rub and chafe the skin, and that foot care is of high priority for carers and students. Often, this is a neglected area, but regular care and assessment by a podiatrist will improve an individual's quality of life.

GROWTH

Adults with Down's syndrome are of characteristically short stature compared with the general population and need to have Down's syndrome-specific growth charts employed to reference growth. Excessive weight-to-height ratios are frequently observed in adults with Down's syndrome, which affect general mobility, especially in the presence of a musculoskeletal abnormality.

ARTHRITIS/ARTHROPATHY

Arthritis refers to the inflammation of a joint which causes pain and swelling of the joint. Arthropathy refers to non-inflammatory disease of a joint, which may have many different causes. There certainly is a higher incidence of joint problems in adults with Down's syndrome, but whether or not there is an increase in the incidence of auto-immune arthritis (such as juvenile rheumatoid arthritis, or JRA) is still being debated in the medical community. One researcher recommended a new condition be named 'arthropathy of Down's syndrome', since the diagnosis of juvenile rheumatoid arthritis is a diagnosis of exclusion (i.e. when you make sure that no other disease process is causing the arthritis, then JRA is all you have left). Most researchers, however, are willing to diagnose JRA in children and teens with Down's syndrome if the specific criteria are met. The treatment of arthritis in people with Down's syndrome is the same as in people without Down's syndrome.

If the joint pains are not inflammatory in origin, then the most likely cause in people with Down's syndrome is the hypermobility of the joints. Other causes may also include psoriasis and gout. Referral to a specialist in arthritis and arthropathies, called a rheumatologist, would be beneficial.

Other causes of articular pain may include psoriasis with associated arthritis, and gout – a disease causing excruciating pain due to deposition of uric acid crystals within synovial joints.

BONES

A small number of studies have indicated that bone density in adults with Down's syndrome is lower than in the general population, thus increasing the risk for osteoporosis in adulthood, especially of the spine. It is not yet known whether supplemental calcium intake will increase bone density in adults with Down's syndrome. Bone density has not yet been studied in children with Down's syndrome. Regardless, there is no evidence that children with Down's syndrome have more broken bones, and likewise there is no evidence that bones in children or adults with Down's syndrome take longer to mend.

COELIAC DISEASE

Adults with Down's syndrome are at a higher risk of developing coeliac disease than the general population. Coeliac disease arises as a result of an allergic autoimmune reaction to gluten – a nitrogenous component of wheat, barley and rye. The lining of the small bowel becomes damaged, causing microscopic anatomical (histological) changes, including flattening of the intestinal villi. As a result, the small bowel becomes unable to absorb water and nutrients. Consequently, individuals with coeliac disease have regular loose bowel movements, which are bulky and foul smelling, and they have diminished appetite (anorexia) and weight loss. Impaired nutrition can affect haemoglobin, causing anaemia, reduced bone density (osteoporosis) and alterations in intestinal bacterial population, leading to abdominal distension and contributing to irritable bowel syndrome (IBS).

The main way of diagnosing coeliac disease is through analysing histological changes within a small tissue sample (biopsy) of the duodenum before and after a period of a gluten-free diet. Treatment involves totally removing gluten from the diet through avoiding all wheat, barley, oat and rye products. In many cases, relief of the symptoms is quickly appreciated – the older the sufferer, the longer the symptoms take to come under control. Coeliac disease is a long-standing (chronic) condition, although there are frequently periods of apparent total recovery (remission), during which time adherence to the dietary regime, which should include vitamin and iron supplements, continues to be necessary.

SKIN CONDITIONS

Atopic dermatitis is the presence of red, scaly, itchy skin. It is most likely to appear on the cheeks, behind the ears, behind the knees and in the elbow creases. Treatment is with steroid creams and oral antihistamines. This is an irritating condition, which needs to be managed by carers to prevent pain and discomfort for those individuals affected.

Seborrhea is a similar condition, but usually greasy and scaly, and appearing on the scalp and eyebrows. Dandruff shampoos or shampoos with either tar compounds or salicylates are used to treat seborrhea of the scalp. Occasionally, antifungal preparations may be useful. This condition can affect an individual's sense of worth and self-esteem, so needs to be treated seriously.

Hyperkeratosis is very thick skin and, in adults with Down's syndrome, occurs on the palms and soles of the feet. Treatment is only tried if the hyperkeratosis appears to bother the person with it, and consists of creams with salicyclic acid or a pumice stone. Hyperkeratosis of the feet can be decreased by wearing comfortable shoes.

Syringomas are benign skin tumours that arise from sweat ducts. They look like very small multiple raised nodules on the skin, with varying degrees of yellowish colour. They are most often seen on the eyelids, neck and chest. Syringomas occur twice as often in females as in males. These do not require treatment, but they can be removed by lasers, shaving or scooping out with a curette.

Elastosis perforans serpiginosa is a disorder of the elastic tissue of the skin, causing deep-red raised lesions to appear in a linear or a circular pattern. These tend to occur on the back and sides of the neck, but may also be seen on the chin, cheeks, arms and knees. These occur in males four times as often as in females. These may last for well over 10 years before going away on their own. Liquid nitrogen is the best current treatment, but this condition has a high rate of recurrence.

Vitiligo is a loss of pigmentation of the skin in well-defined areas. It may occur anywhere on the body and at any age. Vitiligo is not a common problem in adults with Down's syndrome, but is still more common than in the general population. The cause is unknown, but it may be caused by auto-antibodies destroying melanocytes, which are cells in the skin that produce pigment.

Acanthosis nigrans is an increase in pigmentation. The darker skin is also slightly elevated and scaly, often with the appearance of dirt that won't wash off. One large study in Spain reported that out of 51 adults with Down's syndrome, 26 had acanthosis nigrans. This condition most often appears on the back of the neck, the hands and the groin. While acanthosis nigrans has been associated with type II diabetes mellitus, none of the affected adults with Down's syndrome with acanthosis nigrans in the Spanish study had evidence of diabetes.

Chelitis is the presence of fissures and red, scaly skin at the corners of the mouth and lips. This is usually due to moisture collecting at the corners of the mouth, but can also be complicated by infection from bacteria or the yeast *Candida*. The application of a mild steroid cream is useful, along with treating infection when present.

Scabies is an infection of the skin caused by a microscopic mite. For reasons unknown, this infection is a common problem in adults with Down's syndrome and tends to be a worse infection than in the general population. The mite is transmitted by skin-to-skin contact. The rash is extremely itchy and typically appears as small, raised red dots. These dots can appear in lines (the mites burrowing under the skin), but are more often seen in the webs between fingers, around the waist, on the buttocks and around the bra line in females. If the affected person scratches the rash a lot, it can develop a secondary bacterial infection. Scabies usually responds to permethrin cream with a one-time application.

Alopecia (hair loss) is common in both men and women with Down's syndrome. *Alopecia areata* is the term used to describe patchy hair loss, which is not due to infection or drugs. The bald patches have distinct borders, with no hair thinning in other areas of the scalp. Alopecia totalis can also occur. Rarely, hair loss can occur all over the body; this is known as alopecia universalis. Once again, an autoimmune process is thought to be responsible for these conditions, with antibodies being specifically manufactured against hair follicles. Alopecia areata is more common in adults with Down's syndrome, occurring in 5–9 per cent of this population (compared with 1–2 per cent of the general population). A gene implicated in the cause of alopecia areata has been found on the 21st chromosome. There is no cure at present for alopecia; treatment is currently aimed at helping hair re-growth, but it cannot stop the spread of hair loss. The first line of treatment for adults is injection of corticosteroids into the bald spots, with the goal of suppressing the immune reaction causing hair loss. Re-growth can be seen in 4–8 weeks, and treatment is repeated every 4–6 weeks up to a maximum of 6 months. The application of steroid creams is ineffective. There has been some success with hair re-growth with topical applications of minoxidil and anthralin. There are newer agents being tried in clinical studies, such as diphenyl-cyclopropenone and dinitrochlorobenzene, but are not yet commercially available.

CARDIAC (HEART) DEFECTS

Defects within the heart of adults with Down's syndrome are common. Abnormal embryological cardiac development can result in cardiac structural defects. Between 40 and 50 per cent of babies with Down's syndrome have congenital heart defects (Tubman et al. 1991), including atrial and ventricular septal abnormalities, in which blood is inappropriately shunted through structural defects in the atria or ventricles, respectively. The shunting of the blood reduces the effectiveness of the oxygenation function of the blood, resulting in fatigue and cyanosis. Cyanosis can be seen when the skin of the extremities and the mucous membranes turn a dusky blue colour and are cold to the touch. Central cyanosis is seen in the tongue and the lips turn blue, as arterial blood becomes deplete.

Many adults with Down's syndrome have incompetent mitral valves caused by weakening of the valve subsequent to the cardiac infection sub-acute bacterial endocarditis and, as such, require prophylactic preventative antibiotic therapy for dental investigation, as the infective agent can easily gain access to the body through a cut within the mouth. As the student or carer, it is essential that you ensure antibiotics are taken by an adult with Down's syndrome prior to dental treatment, where this is necessary.

Patent ductus arteriosis occurs as the embryonic duct connecting the aorta and pulmonary artery fails to close, resulting in inefficient blood passage throughout the body. Many of these congenital cardiac defects are surgically reversible but rely upon early detection. A high level of clinical suspicion about the presence of cardiac abnormalities must exist for all children with Down's syndrome. Structural defects may well only be symptomatic later in life and missed if echocardiograms have not been utilised in the diagnostic process. It is recommended that screening echocardiograms are employed in the early adulthood of all people with Down's syndrome. Early corrective intervention is essential to minimise the chance of secondary pulmonary disease occurring.

DENTAL

Most adults with Down's syndrome have a compromised immune system and are prone to general infections and have an extremely high incidence of teeth (periodontal), gum (gingival) and mouth (oral) infections. Mouth breathing is common, causing dry mouths (xerostomia). Hypotonia of the muscles associated with eating reduces the effectiveness of chewing (mastication) and with xerostomia can cause bad breath (halitosis). In adults with Down's syndrome, the teeth roots are shorter and less securely embedded, resulting in frequent premature tooth loss.

Good dental hygiene is therefore a requirement when supporting and caring for adults with Down's syndrome, and includes caring for the tongue and gums, even if the person has few or no teeth. Advice should be sought from the dentist or dental hygienist as to the use of dental tape or floss, as it may not be suitable if the person has congenital heart defects, due to the risk of infection entering the bloodstream from small cuts in the gum.

RESPIRATORY DISORDERS

Respiratory disorders are common in adults with Down's syndrome, with the underlying pathology often multifactorial. Structural and functional anomalies such as hypotonia and small lower airway volume can, for example, combine with cardiac defects, excessive mucus secretion and collection in the upper airways to confound accurate diagnosis. As with many adults with learning disabilities, especially those living within communal settings, gastro-oesophageal reflux (GORD) caused by the bacterium *Helicobacter pylori* is very common, causing significant discomfort from gastritis. Sleep disturbance caused by frequent intermittent periods of breathing cessation (sleep apnoea) is common in adults with Down's syndrome and needs investigating to enable an accurate clinical picture of respiratory disturbance from which a diagnostic pathway can be established.

BLOOD CELLS

Larger-than-normal red blood cells (macrocytosis) are common in adults with Down's syndrome, with a microscopic picture revealing an abnormally high mean cell volume (MCV) – a presentation often otherwise seen in bloods from people who habitually imbibe excessive amounts of alcohol.

There are also functional defects of white blood cells in adults with Down's syndrome. White blood cells in adults with Down's syndrome have a decreased response to infection, and a decreased killing ability of microorganisms.

THYROID DISORDERS

Thyroid dysfunction is common in adults with Down's syndrome, with a steady decline in thyroid function increasing with age. Both hypo- and hyper-thyroidism can occur in adults with Down's syndrome, although hypothyroidism is much more common and often caused through an autoimmune process whereby the immunological defence system targets its own body tissues and organs.

Hypothyroidism is caused by a deficiency of thyroxine – a naturally occurring hormone, secreted by the thyroid gland. It is more commonly known as an 'underactive' thyroid. It occurs because the thyroxin gland stops making sufficient thyroxine. Typical symptoms include putting on weight, increasing tiredness and lethargy, constipation and generalised aches and pains (British Thyroid Foundation 2005a). Table 8.2 outlines further clinical features.

The clinical picture of an adult with Down's syndrome suffering from hypothyroidism can be similar to those of both depression and dementia, and careful assessment is required to aid the correct diagnosis and follow-on treatment. This similarity of presenting symptoms is known as differential diagnosis, and therefore careful investigation and diagnosis are needed. Indeed,

Table 8.2. Clinical features of hypothyroidism

- Hearing difficulties
- Facial puffiness
- Husky voice
- Weight gain
- Intolerance of cold
- Hair loss
- Dry skin
- Slow pulse rate
- Constipation
- Lethargy
- Apathy, mental dullness

Table 8.3. Clinical features of hyperthyroidism

- Anxiety
- Irritability
- Palpitations
- Weight loss
- Heat intolerance
- Increased sweating
- Fine tremor
- Menstrual disturbance
- Increased pulse rate
- Warm, sweaty skin
- Diarrhoea
- Retracted eyelids – making the eyes look out-standing

Dennis (2000), representing the Down's Syndrome Association, advises that because of this differential diagnosis, regular blood tests should be carried out on adults with Down's syndrome to assess their thyroid function. It also recommends that carers be alert to the possibility of the thyroid gland slowing down and report these concerns to their GP or learning disability team.

Hyperthyroidism is more usually known as 'overactive thyroid'. The thyroid gland makes too much thyroxine, resulting in some of the following symptoms: noticeable weight loss coupled with an increase in appetite, inability to sleep, restlessness and irritability, palpitations and sweating (British Thyroid Foundation 2005b). Table 8.3 outlines further clinical features.

DEMENTIA

Dementia is a diagnostic term for a collection of illnesses characterised by a global impairment of cognition with normal levels of consciousness. Alzheimer's disease is one type of dementia and is particularly common in adults with Down's syndrome. Many adults with Down's syndrome over the age of 35 years will display signs and symptoms of Alzheimer's disease, such as personality changes, decline in daily living skills, cognitive decline, incontinence, deterioration in memory – initially short-term but, with disease progression, there is virtual total memory loss and the possible occurrence of seizure activity.

A seizure is an alteration in motor, sensory or psychological function attributed to a disordered electrical discharge in the brain. Epilepsy is diagnosed when there is a tendency for recurrent seizures and relies upon accurate and detailed descriptions from the adult with the symptoms and the carers. Most adults with epilepsy will have their symptoms controlled within a medication regime, which will include anticonvulsant therapy. Some lifestyle changes may be required, which will be informed through a comprehensive risk-assessment process balanced with the need to enjoy life to its fullest.

When other physical diagnoses have been ruled out and Alzheimer's disease is suspected, a baseline dementia assessment such as the Dementia Questionnaire for Persons with Mental Retardation (DMR) can be completed. Diagnosis of dementia is based on a decline in functioning over time. Therefore, to ensure a reliable diagnosis, the DMR assessment needs periodic re-tests, to estimate the rate of cognitive decline and ensure that the treatment package is appropriately tailored to meet changing needs. Acetyl cholinesterase-inhibiting drugs (such as Aricept) can be beneficial for some individuals (British Medical Association and the Royal Pharmaceutical Society 2005). The National Institute for Health and Clinical Excellence (NICE) recommended (in January 2001) the use of such drugs under various conditions, including the diagnosis being obtained at a specialist clinic and the patient's being regularly assessed after the maintenance dose is established. The use of drugs can show some possible efficacy in the treatment; early detection can allow appropriate management strategies to be implemented and can also assist in proactively planning for future services to support such individuals. However, it is also important to investigate for treatable conditions which may mimic dementia, such as thyroid disorders, space-occupying lesions (such as brain tumours), neurological conditions and psychological or psychiatric conditions.

As the carer or student, you need to be aware of gradual changes that may show a decline in the memory of the service user whom you are supporting. Signs that need noting include:

- short-term memory loss
- confusion
- apathy
- decline in normal skills
- becoming withdrawn and exhibiting anti-social behaviour
- development of, or increase in, epileptic seizures
- shortfall of road sense.

(Down's Syndrome Association 2006)

SENSORY IMPAIRMENTS

There is a high incidence of eye (ocular) disorders amongst adults with Down's syndrome. Problems with the passage of light rays through the eye (refractive errors), a loss of transparency of the crystalline lens (cataracts), increased pressure within the eye (glaucoma) and squints (strabismus) are all common and may be present from an early age. In some adults with Down's syndrome, a corneal outgrowth (keratoconus) can occur, which, if left untreated, may lead to total blindness. Repeated infection of the margins of the eyelids (blepharitis) and of the membrane covering the front of the eye (conjunctivitis) is again very common in this population. It therefore follows that as the carer or student supporting adults with Down's syndrome it is essential to have good personal care and regular eye checks should form part of annual screening assessments, which will optimise personal health outcomes.

A majority of people with Down's syndrome have a range of significant hearing impairments. Causes can be associated with the auditory nerve (sensorineural), stifling of the sound waves entering the auditory apparatus (conductive) or a mixture of both. The main cause of conductive loss is persistent middle-ear infection (otitis media), often with a discharge (effusion), commonly known as glue ear. In adults with Down's syndrome, this may be a predominantly recurring problem, and they will need frequent monitoring, as hearing loss could be significant (Dennis 2000). Adults with Down's syndrome have anatomically distinct narrow ear canals and this frequently causes a build-up of earwax (cerumen), which affects the hearing. In addition to obvious difficulties in daily living and education, hearing impairment should be considered within the assessment process for dementia and for mood and behaviour disorders.

CONCLUSION

This chapter has briefly examined a range of health issues with particular emphasis upon adults with Down's syndrome. To have 'syndrome-specific' biophysical knowledge should never be avoided for fear of 'medicalising' the support of people with learning disabilities. Effective communication and information sharing are central to effectively meeting the health needs of adults with learning disabilities (Mencap 2004). Medical terminology needs be embraced and understood to support the advocacy and empowerment of our society's most vulnerable citizens – knowledge is, after all, power.

REFERENCES

British Medical Association and the Royal Pharmaceutical Society (2005) *British National Formulary*, London.
British Thyroid Foundation (2005a) *Fact Sheet: Hypothyroidism* (*Underactive Thyroid*), Wetherby, available online at *www.btf-thyroid.org*.
British Thyroid Foundation (2005b) *Fact Sheet: Hyperthyroidism* (*Overactive Thyroid*), Wetherby, available online at *www.btf-thyroid.org*.

Casey, A. T., O'Brien, M., Kumar, V., Hayward, R. D. & Crockard, H. A. (1995) 'Don't Twist my Child's Head Off: Latrogenic Cervical Dislocation', *British Medical Journal*, **311**(4): 1212–13.

Davidson, R. G. (1988) 'Atlantoaxial Instability in Individuals with Down's Syndrome: A Fresh Look at the Evidence', *Paediatrics*, **81**: 857–65.

Dennis, J. (2000) *1. Thyroid Disorder among People with Down's Syndrome: Notes for Parents and Carers*, London, Down's Syndrome Association.

Department of Health (1995) *Cervical Spine: Inotability in People with Down's Syndrome*, CMO update 7, p. 4.

Department of Health (2001) *Valuing People: A New Strategy for Learning Disabilities for the 21st Century*, London, Department of Health.

Down's Syndrome Association (2006) *Leaflet 15: Promoting Health in People with Down's Syndrome*, London.

Frey, L., Szalda-Petree, A., Traci, M. A. & Seekins, T. (2001) 'Prevention of Secondary Health Conditions in Adults with Developmental Disabilities: A Review of the Literature', *Disability and Rehabilitation*, **23**(9): 361–9.

Hollins, S., Attard, T., von Fraunhofer, N., McGuigan, S. & Sedgewick, P. (1998) 'Mortality in People with Learning Disability: Risks, Causes and Death Certification Findings in London', *Developmental Medicine and Child Neurology*, **40**: 50–6, also in National Patient Safety Agency (2004) *Understanding the Patient Safety Issues for People with Learning Disabilities*.

Kerr, M. (1998) 'Primary Healthcare and Health Gains for People with a Learning Disability', *Tizard Learning Disability Review*, **4**: 6–14.

Martin, D. M., Roy, A. & Wells, M. B. (1997) 'Health Gain through Health Checks: Improving Access to Primary Healthcare for People with Intellectual Disability', *Journal of Intellectual Disability Research*, **41**(5): 401–8.

Mencap (2004) *Treat Me Right! Better Healthcare for People with a Learning Disability*, Mencap.

Tubman, T. R. J., Sheilds, M. G., Craig, B. Q., Mullholland, H. C. & Nevin, N. C. (1991) 'Congenital Heart Disease in Down's Syndrome; 2 Year Prospective Early Screening Study', *British Medical Journal*, **302**: 1425–7.

Van Schrojenstein Lantman-de Valk, H. M., Metsemakers, J. F., Haveman, M. J. & Crebolder, H. F. (2000) 'Health Problems in People with Intellectual Disability in General Practice: A Comparative Study', *Family Practice*, **17**(S): 405–7.

9 Legislation and Learning Disabilities

MALCOLM McIVER

KEY POINTS

- Adults with learning disabilities are, for the most part, subject to the same laws as every other member of society.
- The term 'mental impairment' is a term used in law – in the Mental Health Act 1983, this is, in effect, learning disability.
- Learning disability alone is not sufficient justification to apply the Mental Health Act; the definitions of both mental impairment and severe mental impairment include the condition of 'abnormally aggressive or seriously irresponsible conduct'.
- Legislation at the dawn of the twenty-first century strives to protect.

INTRODUCTION

'There is no investigator who denies the fearful role played by mental deficiency in the production of vice, crime and delinquency. Not all criminals are feeble-minded, but all feeble-minded are at least a potential criminal.'

(Terman 1916)

So wrote Lewis Terman, an eminent and much respected cognitive psychologist, at the beginning of the twentieth century. Today, his words appear shocking and would be rightly condemned as bigoted. Yet, for much of the last century, and the years that preceded it, the above sentiments were commonplace throughout Western society. Many young women who had a child outside of marriage were often diagnosed as 'moral defectives' and immediately dispatched to an institution, where, quite often, they would remain for the rest of their lives. In some instances, simply to be suspected of engaging in sexual activity outside of marriage was sufficient to deprive a person of their liberty (Wilkey, in Chapter 10 in this book, discusses these issues further). Although less likely to be diagnosed as morally defective, unless suspected of homosexual activity, men with a learning disability fared little better. Conviction of a minor criminal offence that would normally incur a fine for most offenders often resulted in detention without limit in a mental institution. Such was the public's fear of people with learning disabilities that the slightest indiscretion often resulted in what, in effect, was a life sentence.

At this point, you may be asking yourself what has any of this to do with legislation in the twenty-first century? Well, the answer is that none of the above could or would have happened if the legislation of the day had not permitted it. Legislation is the barometer of society's attitude towards those they legislate for, and those they legislate against. So what does today's legislation say about people with learning disabilities in the twenty-first century?

THE LEGISLATION

People with learning disabilities are, for the most part, subject to the same laws as every other member of society. There are, however, several pieces of legislation that are of particular interest to people with learning disabilities and their carers. Throughout this chapter, four key pieces of legislation that reflect society's current perceptions of people with learning disabilities will be explored. This exploration will, by necessity, be quite brief; an in-depth exploration of the legislation cannot be accommodated in a single chapter. However, the salient points will be discussed.

At first sight, the study of learning disability legislation may appear daunting to those embarking upon it for the first time. The Mental Health Act 1983 alone contains 10 parts and 149 sections, but do not despair. Unless you are intending to pursue a legal career, most readers of this chapter will not require an in-depth knowledge of every part of every section of every act. Therefore, to ease your introduction into the world of legislation, only those sections that are immediately relevant to people with learning disabilities and their carers will be discussed. That is not to say that those sections that are not discussed here are irrelevant, but rather that they can and *should* be explored at a later date. The order in which they are discussed is not intended to be a reflection of any judgement upon them, but simply reflects the chronological order in which these acts became law.

THE MENTAL HEALTH ACT 1983

The introduction of the Mental Health Act in 1983, replacing the previous 1959 Act, was hailed by its proponents as a radical piece of legislation that embraced the principles of civil liberties, whilst affording protection to service users and the public at large. The then Chairman of the Royal College of

Psychiatrists Working Party described the new act as 'an event in the history of mental health care of the greatest importance' (Bluglass 1983). Although it is now more than two decades since the act was passed, the legislation remains in force at the time of writing. Readers should be aware, however, that amendments to the act are pending. So what does the Mental Health Act 1983 contain?

PARTS OF THE ACT

As with all legislation, the act is arranged in parts. These parts are:

- Part I: Application of Act
- Part II: Compulsory Admission to Hospitals and Guardianship
- Part III: Patients Concerned in Criminal Proceedings or under Sentence
- Part IV: Consent to Treatment
- Part V: Mental Health Review Tribunals
- Part VI: Removal and Return of Patients within the United Kingdom
- Part VII: Management of Property and Affairs of Patients
- Part VIII: Miscellaneous Functions of Local Authorities and the Secretary of State
- Part IX: Offences
- Part X: Miscellaneous and Supplementary

It can be seen from a brief examination of the above headings that the act is primarily concerned with the admission, detention and treatment of those 'patients' that require it. (The word 'patient' is used here because that was the term employed within the act and was the language of the day.) The first part that is of key interest is Part I, for it is here that those people to whom the act is applied are defined.

PART I: APPLICATION OF THE ACT

Section 1 of Part I provides a *legal,* rather than a medical, definition of the types of mental health problems that the Mental Health Act 1983 is intended to cover, and identifies the scope of the act:

'1.–(1) The provisions of this Act shall have effect with respect to the reception, care and treatment of mentally disordered patients, the management of their property and other related matters.'

Mental disorder is divided into four types:

(1) Severe Mental Impairment,
(2) Mental Impairment,

(3) Psychopathic Disorder, and
(4) Mental Illness.

The two that are of particular interest to those working in the field of learning disabilities are mental impairment and severe mental impairment, further defined thus:

> 'Severe mental impairment means a state of arrested or incomplete development of mind which includes severe impairment of intelligence and social functioning and is associated with abnormally aggressive or seriously irresponsible conduct on the part of the person concerned and "severely mentally impaired" shall be construed accordingly; Mental impairment means a state of arrested or incomplete development of mind (not amounting to severe mental impairment) which includes significant impairment of intelligence and social functioning and is associated with abnormally aggressive or seriously irresponsible conduct on the part of the person concerned and "mentally impaired" shall be construed accordingly.'

It can be seen from these definitions that 'mental impairment' is, in effect, learning disability. However, learning disability alone is not sufficient justification to apply the act, as the definitions of both 'mental impairment' and 'severe mental impairment' include the condition of 'abnormally aggressive or seriously irresponsible conduct'. So, the act only applies to adults with learning disabilities who also exhibit abnormally aggressive or seriously irresponsible behaviour. In practice, this represents a tiny proportion of adults with learning disabilities.

PART II: COMPULSORY ADMISSION TO HOSPITAL

Part II of the act contains the sections which set out the criteria for compulsorily detaining people in hospital. An interesting feature of the act is that compulsory detention may not require any judicial involvement, unlike in many other countries (including Scotland), where compulsory detention requires a judge's approval. In England and Wales, the decision to detain can be taken by doctors, social workers and, in certain circumstances, nurses. The most common civil sections of the act under which patients are compulsorily admitted to a hospital are sections 2, 3 and 4. There are other sections of the act that permit detention, but those will be explored later.

Section 2

Section 2 provides the authority for someone to be detained in hospital for up to 28 days for assessment purposes only. The grounds for the application, as stated in the act, are that the person:

(1) is suffering from mental disorder of a nature or degree which warrants the detention of the patient in a hospital for assessment (or for assessment followed by medical treatment) for at least a limited period; *and*
(2) he ought to be so detained in the interests of his own health or safety or with a view to the protection of other persons.

This section is most often applied when someone is compulsorily admitted to hospital for the first time, or if there has been a considerable gap since the last admission. Application to detain someone under section 2 of the act requires two medical recommendations. One of those recommendations must be made by an approved doctor, which, for the purposes of the act, is defined as a doctor with 'special experience in the diagnosis or treatment of mental disorder'. This is usually a consultant or senior registrar, whilst the second medical recommendation most often is made by the person's general practitioner (GP).

Although the act does not prohibit an application for a second section 2 detention immediately after the 28-day period has ended, in practice, this does not occur. The 28-day period is intended solely to provide time to assess the individual's condition. If continued detention is required, then section 3 is normally applied.

Section 3

Section 3 provides the authority for someone to be detained in hospital for *up to* 6 months for treatment. As with section 2, an application to apply section 3 requires two medical recommendations. The grounds for the application, as stated in the act, are that the person:

(1) is suffering from mental illness, severe mental impairment, psychopathic disorder or mental impairment and his mental disorder is of a nature or degree which make it appropriate for him to receive medical treatment in a hospital; *and*
(2) in the case of psychopathic disorder or mental impairment, such treatment is likely to alleviate or prevent a deterioration of his condition; *and*
(3) it is necessary for the health or safety of the patient or for the protection of other persons that he should receive such treatment and it cannot be provided unless he is detained under this Section.

This section is typically used when a section 2 has expired, and extended treatment is required. It is also commonly used where someone with a mental disorder is well known to the hospital. This enables a firm treatment plan, rather than open-ended assessment, to commence early in the period of detention. If treatment is still required after the initial 6 months, this section can be renewed for a further 6 months and then for 12 months at a time. Although uncommon in practice, it is worth noting that a section 3 cannot normally be imposed if the nearest relative objects.

Section 4

Section 4 is an emergency admission for assessment for up to 72 hours and is intended for situations in which if it were not for the extreme urgency, a section 2 would normally be applied. As this is an emergency admission, only *one* medical recommendation is required, preferably by a doctor who is familiar with the individual. The grounds for the application are the same as for section 2. However, in addition, it must be stated that:

(1) it is of urgent necessity for the patient to be admitted and detained under section 2, *and*
(2) that compliance with the usual section 2 requirements (that is, getting a second medical recommendation) would involve 'undesirable delay'.

If a second medical recommendation is made before the 72 hours expire, section 4 is effectively converted into a section 2, permitting the individual to be detained for up to 28 days.

Sections 5(2) and 5(4)

Although not commonly used, the following sections are worth noting. Section 5(2), known as the Doctors' Holding Power, permits a doctor to legally detain a voluntary patient for up to 72 hours. This section is applied where it is believed that the patient is a danger to himself or others and that, in the opinion of the doctor, detention under the act is necessary. The 72 hours are intended to permit further assessment to be undertaken and, if necessary, to arrange a section 2 or section 3 admission. If no further sections are applied after the 72 hours, the patient is then free to take his/her discharge if s/he so wishes.

Section 5(4), known as the Nurses' Holding Power, is used even less commonly than section 5(2). However, it is essential that those nurses qualified to exercise this power (Registered Mental Nurse or Registered Learning Disability Nurse) are familiar with the section. As with the doctors, the holding power of section 5(4) permits voluntary patients to be legally detained; unlike section 5(4), however, the period of detention is only 6 hours. The grounds for the application are that it appears to the nurse:

(1) that the patient is suffering from mental disorder to such a degree that it is necessary for his health or safety or for the protection of others for him to be immediately restrained from leaving the hospital; *and*

(2) that it is not practicable to secure the immediate attendance of a medical practitioner for the purpose of furnishing a report under section 5(2).

The nurse simply has to record in writing that the conditions are met. This written record has to be conveyed to the hospital managers as soon as possible. The patient can then be prevented from leaving the ward pending the arrival of the doctor, who could, if necessary, impose a section 5(2). If the doctor imposes a section 5(2), the 72-hour period of the section 5(2) starts from the time of the original section 5(4) report by the nurse.

PART III: PATIENTS CONCERNED IN CRIMINAL PROCEEDINGS OR UNDER SENTENCE

Unlike the sections in Part II, Part III deals with compulsory detention that does involve the judiciary.

Section 35

Section 35 allows a court to send a person to hospital for 28 days for a report to be prepared on his/her mental condition, instead of remanding the person to prison. This period can be extended by the court for not more than 28 days at a time, up to a maximum of 12 weeks. The purpose of section 35 is assessment and preparation of a report only. Prior to imposing a section 35, the court must be satisfied that:

(1) there is reason to suspect that the accused person has at least one of the four types of mental disorder, on the basis of evidence supplied by an approved doctor *and*
(2) it would not be practicable for the necessary report to be prepared if the person were allowed bail *and*
(3) a specific hospital is willing and able to admit the person within 7 days.

The imposition of a section 35, however, is restricted to those persons who fulfil the above criteria and:

- have been charged with an offence which could lead to a jail term and
- will be before a Crown Court, but not yet tried/convicted *or*
- will have been convicted by a Magistrates' Court *or*
- will be before a Magistrates' Court, but not have been convicted, *and* either: the court is satisfied that that the person did what they are accused of doing *or*
- the person agrees to a section 35 remand being made.

The exception to this is when a person has *been convicted* of murder, in which case the court has to impose a sentence of life imprisonment in all cases.

It should be noted that although the individuals are detained in a hospital, they remain under the control of the court. They cannot be discharged, nor do they have a right of appeal. People remanded under section 35 do not have to accept medication or other treatment against their will.

Section 36

Where compulsory treatment may be required, the court has the option of applying section 36. This, however, can only be imposed by a Crown Court, *not* a Magistrates' Court. This section permits the court to send a person to hospital, for an initial period of 28 days, for treatment, rather than remanding him/her to prison. This period can be extended by the court but for not more than 28 days at a time, and only up to a maximum of 12 weeks. As with section 35, the court must be satisfied that:

(1) that the accused person has mental illness or severe mental impairment, on the basis of evidence supplied by two doctors (at least one of whom must be approved under Section 12) *and*
(2) that a specific hospital is willing and able to admit the person within 7 days.

The person concerned must be appearing before a Crown Court and charged with an offence which could lead to imprisonment. As with section 35, section 36 cannot be used when a person has *been convicted* of murder; the court has to impose a sentence of life imprisonment in all cases. Similarly, s/he remains under the control of the court. S/he cannot be discharged, may be treated compulsorily and has no right of appeal. However, it should be noted that unlike section 35, it cannot be imposed upon someone who has only *been accused and not convicted* of murder.

Section 37

Section 37 allows a court to send a person to hospital for treatment when otherwise the outcome might have been a prison sentence. The order is *instead of* imprisonment, a fine or probation. The order is initially for a period of 6 months, beginning on the date of the order. It can, however, be renewed for a further 6 months, and then annually. Prior to imposing the order, the court must be satisfied that:

(1) the person has at least one of the four types of mental disorder, supported with evidence from two doctors, *and*
(2) the mental disorder is of such a degree or nature that makes it appropriate for the person to be detained in hospital for medical treatment (and, in the case of psychopathic disorder or mental impairment, that the treat-

ment is likely to alleviate or prevent a deterioration of the person's condition) *and*
(3) that making a section 37 order is the most suitable way of dealing with the person, bearing in mind all relevant matters *and*
(4) that a specific hospital is willing and able to admit the person within 28 days.

Furthermore, the detained individual *must* have:

(1) been convicted by a Crown Court of an offence which could be punished with imprisonment (except in the case of murder) *or*
(2) been convicted by a Magistrates' Court of an offence which could be punished with imprisonment *or*
(3) been convicted, but may be before a Magistrates' Court charged with an offence which could lead to imprisonment if the person were convicted.

It is notable that in some circumstances, the court can still impose a section 37 order, even without a conviction, if it is satisfied that the person did what she or he is accused of doing and the person has mental illness or severe mental impairment.

PART V: MENTAL HEALTH REVIEW TRIBUNALS

The Mental Health Act 1983 contains no fewer than 149 sections; the above sections are only those that new practitioners and students of mental health legislation need to familiarise themselves with *initially*. Whilst it is not possible to explore the remaining sections here, readers are advised to acquaint themselves with the entire act, although it should be reiterated that amendments to the act are pending. There is, however, one other section that readers do need to be aware of – section 66.

Section 66

Section 66 of the Mental Health Act 1983 put in place the legislation required to create the Mental Health Review Tribunals. There is a Tribunal for each of the National Health Service Regions in England, with a single one just for Wales. Each Tribunal consists of medical members, legal members and lay members. Every member is appointed by the Lord Chancellor, although the appointment of the lay and medical members is undertaken following consultation with the Secretary of State, under the guidance of the Department of Constitutional Affairs. The purpose of the Mental Health Review Tribunals is to hear appeals against detention, *for those sections in which appeals are permitted*, from either the individual who is detained or his/her nearest relative. The act also imposes a duty upon hospital managers to automatically refer cases to the Tribunal where detained individuals eligible to appeal, or their nearest relative, have failed to do so.

Every detained patient whose section permits an appeal is entitled to make one application to the Tribunal for each of the authorised periods of detention. Proceedings are generally formal and often the parties involved will be represented by lawyers. After considering an appeal, there are a number of options available to the Tribunal. It can:

- reject the appeal, in which case the detention order remains in place for the duration of the authorised period, *or*
- reclassify the form of mental disorder on the application, for example it may conclude that a patient is suffering from mental impairment rather than, say, psychopathic disorder, *or*
- direct that a patient be discharged, *or*
- recommend the patient be granted leave of absence, *or*
- direct that the patient be transferred to another hospital, *or*
- transfer into guardianship.

For people with learning disabilities and their carers, the Mental Health Act 1983 is, for the most part, irrelevant. Only those who exhibit abnormally aggressive or seriously irresponsible behaviour will be subject to it. However, for those who are subjected to it, the legislation now looks increasingly dated and fails to reflect current human rights legislation. It is envisaged that the amendments to the act will take into account human rights law and introduce significant new rights and safeguards for patients.

THE DISABILITY DISCRIMINATION ACT 1995

Imagine a world in which the bar staff in a pub shouted 'I don't want your kind in here' as soon as you walked through the door, in which your local cinema barred you because you were a 'health hazard' and large stores turned you away because 'seeing you would upset their regular customers'. Now imagine that there is absolutely nothing you can do about it. You cannot retort 'I know my rights' because you don't have any. You cannot take legal action because no offence has been committed. There is no one to complain to – you simply have to accept it.

Not that many years ago, this was the world as many adults with learning disabilities in the United Kingdom knew it. Yet, amazingly, this was not discrimination. There was no such offence as disability discrimination. That, however, has now changed with the introduction of the Disability Discrimination Act 1995. Introduced in phases between 1996 and 2005, the Disability Discrimination Act is the first piece of legislation to specifically address issues of disability in the United Kingdom since the Chronically Sick and Disabled

Act of 1945, and the first in the United Kingdom to address the discrimination faced by disabled people. With eight Parts and 70 sections, the most important sections of the act for people with learning disabilities are contained in Parts I–V.

PART I: DISABILITY

Part I, section 1 defines disability as 'a person has a disability for the purposes of this Act if he has a physical or mental impairment which has a substantial and long-term adverse effect on his ability to carry out normal day-to-day activities'. For the purposes of the act, 'long-term' means that the person has had the disability for more than 12 months and/or it is expected to continue for 12 months or more, whilst 'normal day-to-day activities' include:

- mobility
- manual dexterity
- physical coordination
- speech, hearing or eyesight
- continence
- the ability to lift, carry or move ordinary objects
- memory, or the ability to concentrate, learn or understand
- being able to recognise physical danger.

Clearly, this broad definition encompasses those with a learning disability, and, as such, they are entitled to the protection that this legislation affords. So what protection does it afford?

PART II: EMPLOYMENT

Part II, section 4 of the act, which places a duty on employers not to discriminate against disabled employees or applicants for employment, came into force on 2 December 1996. At that time, the act only applied to employers who employed 15 or more employers. However, since October 2004, the legislation now applies to all employers, regardless of the number of people whom they employ. As a consequence of the act, it is unlawful for employers to treat a disabled person less favourably than a non-disabled person. This includes the recruitment and interviewing of new employees, the terms of employment, such as length of contract and salary, training, promotion, transfers and dismissal procedures. Employers are still able to recruit or promote the most suitable or best equipped candidate for a job but they cannot now reject a candidate or pay him/her less solely on the grounds that s/he is disabled.

Furthermore, section 6(1) of Part II states that 'Where – (a) any arrangements made by or on behalf of an employer, or (b) any physical feature of premises occupied by the employer place the disabled person concerned at a substantial disadvantage in comparison with persons who are not disabled, it is the duty of the employer to take such steps as it is reasonable, in all the circumstances of the case, for him to have to take in order to prevent the arrangements or feature having that effect'.

In effect, this requires employers to make reasonable changes to the workplace or working practices to enable the disabled person to carry out the job, providing these changes do not breach health and safety laws. Examples of reasonable adjustments identified in the act include:

- making adjustments to premises
- allocating some of the disabled person's duties to another person
- altering their working hours
- allowing the disabled person to be absent during working hours for rehabilitation, assessment or treatment
- providing or arranging for training
- modifying equipment
- modifying assessment procedures
- providing a reader or interpreter
- providing supervision.

The duty of the employer to make reasonable adjustments, however, is not absolute and applies only if (a) the disabled person is at a disadvantage, and (b) the adjustments are reasonable. In determining what is reasonable, the employer is entitled to consider the cost in relation to the benefits of any changes. Where the cost of making the change proves prohibitively expensive and/or results in minimum benefit, employers will be able to argue that the adjustments are not reasonable.

This is not the only exemption, as the employment provision in the legislation does not apply to the armed forces, the police service, the fire service and the prison service or to anyone employed onboard ships, aeroplanes or hovercraft.

PART III: DISCRIMINATION IN OTHER AREAS – GOODS, FACILITIES AND SERVICES

Section 19 of Part III, which also came into force in December 1996, places a duty on providers of goods, facilities and services (service providers) not to discriminate against disabled people. The range of different service providers is far too extensive to list here; however, some examples include:

- hotels
- pubs
- shops

- theatres
- churches
- parks
- train stations
- airports
- housing associations and hostels.

Education is, as is public transport, excluded from this, as they are covered in Parts IV and V, respectively. In October 1999, a number of further provisions were enforced which require service providers to make reasonable adjustments to policies, practices and procedures, and to provide auxiliary aids and services.

Under section 20(1) of the act, a service provider is said to have discriminated against a disabled person if '(a) for a reason which relates to the disabled person's disability, he treats him less favourably than he treats or would treat others to whom that reason does not or would not apply; and (b) he cannot show that the treatment in question is justified'.

As a consequence, it is now unlawful for a service provider to:

(1) refuse to provide, or deliberately not provide, a service to a disabled person when it is normally offered to other people;
(2) provide a lower standard of service, or in a worse manner;
(3) provide a service on less favourable terms.

Part III also puts a separate duty on people selling, renting or managing property not to discriminate against disabled people. Where a physical feature makes it unreasonably difficult or impossible for a disabled person to make use of a service provider's services, the provider now has a duty to find a reasonable alternative way of making their service available and, since October 2004, they are required to consider either removing the physical feature, altering it or providing a reasonable means of avoiding it. As with Part II, there is a cost–benefit criterion in determining what is reasonable. However, it is no longer legally acceptable, for example, for a pub, theatre or shop to exclude or limit the access of people with learning disabilities *solely on the grounds of disability* to the services and leisure facilities that most of us take for granted.

PART IV: EDUCATION

Although excluded from Part III of the act ('Provision of Goods, Services and Facilities'), Part IV did recognise the needs of disabled people in relation to education. However, the Special Educational Needs and Disability Act 2001 (SENDA) amended the DDA 1995, imposing new duties for education providers, which came into effect in September 2002. Section 28A(1) states that 'It is unlawful for the body responsible for a school to discriminate against a disabled person – (a) in the arrangements it makes for determining admission to the school as a pupil; (b) in the terms on which it offers to admit him to the school as a pupil; or (c) by refusing or deliberately omitting to accept an application for his admission to the school as a pupil'. Similarly, section 28A(4) states that 'It is unlawful for the body responsible for a school to discriminate against a disabled pupil by excluding him from the school, whether permanently or temporarily'.

As with the earlier parts of the act, the meaning of 'discrimination', in relation to education, is treating an individual with a disability less favourably than others when it cannot be shown that the treatment in question is justified. Under section 28C, it is also considered to be discrimination if an educational provider fails to take 'reasonable' steps to 'ensure that (a) in relation to the arrangements it makes for determining the admission of pupils to the school, disabled persons are not placed at a substantial disadvantage in comparison with persons who are not disabled; and (b) in relation to education and associated services provided for, or offered to, pupils at the school by it, disabled pupils are not placed at a substantial disadvantage in comparison with pupils who are not disabled'.

As a consequence of these amendments, Part IV of the act has now been brought into line with Part III, and providers of education now have a duty to make 'reasonable' adjustments to working practices and premises where existing premises or practices put disabled people at a substantial disadvantage. These might include:

- changing admissions, administrative and examination procedures;
- changing course content, including work placements;
- changing physical features and premises;
- changing teaching arrangements;
- providing additional teaching;
- providing communication and support services;
- offering information in alternative formats;
- training staff.

However, if those adjustments would lower academic standards, then education providers are not compelled to make them. The act also requires all education authorities to prepare an accessibility strategy to:

(a) increase the extent to which disabled pupils can participate in the schools' curriculums,
(b) improve the physical environment of the schools for the purpose of increasing the extent to which disabled pupils are able to take advantage of education and associated services provided or offered by the schools;

(c) improve the delivery to disabled pupils within a reasonable time, and in ways which are determined after taking account of their disabilities and any preferences expressed by them or their parents.

PART V: PUBLIC TRANSPORT

Part V of the 1995 Act did little other than give the government powers to make regulations relating to the design and accessibility of public transport vehicles, such as taxis, buses, coaches, trains and trams at a later date. This paved the way for the Disability Discrimination Act 2005 which identifies minimum standards, and a timetable for the introduction of those standards. However, whilst the 2005 amendment to the act requires public transport operators to ensure that all *new* vehicles, including rail vehicles and newly licensed taxis, are (a) accessible to disabled people, and (b) that disabled people are able to travel in safety and reasonable comfort, the legislation did not take immediate effect. The dates of the introduction of these duties vary according to the type of vehicle:

- Taxis: *new* taxis should now be made accessible. All vehicles should meet the requirements by the year 2012.
- Buses and coaches: all *new* single-decker buses should now be accessible. All double-decker buses should now also be accessible. All vehicles will have to comply with the regulations at a later date.
- Rail vehicles: all *new* rail vehicles that have come into service after 31 December 1998 will have to comply with the regulations.

As with other service providers, transport operators will have to make 'reasonable' adjustments to policies, practices and procedures that discriminate against disabled people and also to provide auxiliary aids and services where they enable or facilitate access. However, it should be noted that even with the legislation, it is likely to be 2020 before all public transport is fully accessible to people with disabilities.

As stated earlier, the above five parts of the Disability Discrimination Act 1995 are likely to be of the most immediate interest to people with learning disabilities, as they identify those areas in which disability discrimination has been outlawed. There is, however, one further part of the act that is worthy of consideration and that is Part VI.

PART VI

Earlier anti-discriminatory legislation (the Sex Discrimination Act 1975 and the Race Relations Act 1976) had created commissions such as the Equal

Opportunities Commission and the Commission for Racial Equality. Part VI of the Disability Discrimination Act 1995, however, created the National Disability Council. Whereas the Commissions can hear complaints and have the power to take action against those found to have acted in a discriminatory manner, the remit of the National Disability Council was to merely advise the Secretary of State on matters 'relevant to the elimination of discrimination against disabled persons'.

For many, this was seen as a major weakness of the legislation, as, in the absence of a Commission, the only course of action open to those who believed that they had been discriminated against was a prohibitively expensive private legal action. However, in response to these criticisms, 4 years after the Disability Discrimination Act came into force, the Government passed the Disability Rights Commission Act 1999, which abolished the National Disability Council and replaced it in 2000 with the Disability Rights Commission. Unlike the earlier Council, whose role was simply to advise government, the remit of the Commission is far more extensive and includes:

- promoting equal opportunities for disabled people in the provision of services;
- providing information and advice to anyone with rights or duties under the act;
- supplying assistance and support to disabled litigants;
- undertaking formal investigations into discrimination and ensuring compliance with the law;
- arranging a conciliation service between service providers and disabled people to help resolve.

More importantly, the Commission can also take offenders to court, where a successful prosecution could result in compensation or an injunction forbidding the offender from repeating the discriminatory behaviour. Whilst it is unlikely that the Disability Discrimination Act will completely eradicate discrimination against people with disabilities, the legislation does give people with learning disabilities the right to access the services and facilities that most of us take for granted, and a means to take action where that right is denied.

THE HUMAN RIGHTS ACT 1998

Introduced in to the United Kingdom in October 2000, the Human Rights Act 1998 did not actually create any new rights for individuals. Nor did it specifically refer to people with learning disabilities. So why is it important? Well, the Human Rights Act enshrined within UK legislation, for the very first time, the articles and protocols found in the European Convention on Human Rights. Quite simply, following the introduction of the act, all UK legislation such as any amendment to the Mental Health Act or any legislation that relates to people with learning disabilities must now comply with the rights contained within the act. Table 9.1 outlines the Articles.

The act is also intended to protect individuals from abuses by the state or the institutions of the state. It is now unlawful for any public authority, such as a health or local authority, to breach the rights set out in the Convention. For example, an adult with a learning disability who has a heart condition is now legally entitled to receive the same *standard* of treatment for that heart condition as any other person with a similar condition. (I specify *standard* of

Table 9.1. An outline of the Human Rights Articles

- **Article 1 of Protocol 1 Protection of Property** Nobody has the right to unlawfully interfere with personal possessions. Every individual has the right to peaceful enjoyment of their possessions.
- **Article 2 of Protocol 1 Right to Education** The right NOT to be denied access to the educational system.
- **Article 3 of Protocol 1 Right to Free Elections** Free and fair elections for parliament must take place by secret ballot.
- **Article 2 The Right to Life** Every individual has the absolute right to life, protected by law.
- **Article 3 The Prohibition of Torture** The right not to be tortured or subjected to treatment that is inhuman or degrading.
- **Article 4 The Prohibition of Slavery or Forced Labour** The right not to be forced into slavery or forced into certain types of labour.
- **Article 5 The Right to Liberty, Personal Freedom and Security** The right NOT to be deprived of freedom (unless suspected or convicted of committing a crime).
- **Article 6 The Right to a Fair Trial** The right to a fair and public hearing by an independent tribunal established by law.
- **Article 7 No Punishment without Law** The right not to be found guilty of offences from actions that were not criminal.
- **Article 8 The Right to Respect for Private and Family Life** To have private family life respected, and private correspondence treated confidentially.
- **Article 9 The Right to Freedom of Thought, Conscience and Religion** The right to hold a broad range of views and religious beliefs.
- **Article 10 The Right to Freedom of Expression** The right to hold opinions and to express views on all subjects.
- **Article 11 Freedom of Assembly and Association** The right to assemble with others in a peaceful way, to peacefully protest, for example, or to form trades unions.
- **Article 12 The Right to Marry** Under this right, national laws will still govern how marriages take place, and the legal age at which people can marry.
- **Article 14 Prohibition of Discrimination** The right not to be treated differently because of race, religion, sex, political views or any other status.

treatment here because decisions on specific treatments are, of course, governed by clinical considerations.) For a hospital or health authority to discriminate on the grounds of learning disability, as sometimes happened in the past, is now a breach of the Human Rights Act. Furthermore, the act should make the process of claiming rights easier. Previously, any individual who believed that his/her rights had been breached had to take his/her case to the European Court of Human Rights in Strasbourg. The cases can now be heard in the United Kingdom, and dealt with by a UK court or tribunal. However, it should be noted that it is not intended that the act be used to bring actions against private individuals. It is still not possible to sue, or, for that matter, be sued by, another for breaking the rights in the Convention.

In essence, the Human Rights Act is designed to affect the way in which public authorities behave, and to ensure that they pay attention to people's rights, ensuring that everyone receives the benefit of the law, regardless of race, ethnicity, religion, gender, mental, physical or learning disability.

MENTAL CAPACITY ACT 2005

The latest and quite possibly most controversial piece of legislation that relates to people with learning disabilities is the Mental Capacity Act 2005. The Mental Incapacity Bill, as it was originally known, received Royal Assent in April 2005 and is expected to come into force in England and Wales in 2007. (Scotland has its own Adults with Incapacity Act 2000.) When it does come into force, it will affect everyone over the age of 16 years whose mental capacity is in doubt, and those who care for them. Mental capacity, in relation to the legislation, refers to the ability of the individual to make a decision about some aspect of his/her life. Although the act is not limited to specific conditions, mental capacity can be affected by many conditions, such as dementia, stroke or mental illness; this legislation will have major implications for a substantial number of people with learning disabilities and their carers. In brief, the stated aim of the act is to provide a statutory framework that will empower and protect vulnerable people who are unable to make their own decisions, and make clear who can take decisions on their behalf and in what situation(s). Individual care plans will have to conform to the principles of the act, demonstrating that service users have either been involved in decisions about their care, or that they have been assessed as lacking the capacity to do so and that the decisions made are in their best interests. In order to ensure that vulnerable people are protected and empowered, the entire act is underpinned by five key principles. Sections 1–4 of the act best illustrate those key principles and will be discussed here. However, readers are advised that there are many more sections to the act (68 in total) which may be of interest to them.

SECTION 1: KEY PRINCIPLES

Part I, section 1 introduces the five key principles that apply throughout the act. These principles are:

(1) A person must be assumed to have capacity unless it is established that he lacks capacity.
(2) A person is not to be treated as unable to make a decision unless all practicable steps to help him to do so have been taken without success.
(3) A person is not to be treated as unable to make a decision merely because he makes an unwise decision.
(4) An act done or decision made under this Act for or on behalf of a person who lacks capacity must be done, or made, in his best interests.
(5) Before the act is done, or the decision is made, regard must be had to whether the purpose for which it is needed can be as effectively achieved in a way that is less restrictive of the person's rights and freedom of action.

SECTION 2: PEOPLE WHO LACK CAPACITY

It can be seen from the very first principle that, similar to the presumption of innocence that underpins criminal legislation in the United Kingdom, it is not the responsibility of individuals to prove their mental capacity but rather that others must prove their incapacity. Section 2 of the act identifies those to whom the act applies and describes people who lack capacity in the following terms:

(1) For the purposes of this act, a person lacks capacity in relation to a matter if at the material time he is unable to make a decision for himself in relation to the matter because of an impairment of, or a disturbance in the functioning of, the mind or brain.
(2) It does not matter whether the impairment or disturbance is permanent or temporary.
(3) A lack of capacity cannot be established merely by reference to –
    (a) a person's age or appearance, or
    (b) a condition of his, or an aspect of his behaviour, which might lead others to make unjustified assumptions about his capacity.

In effect, this means that the assessment of an individual's mental capacity is time- and issue-specific. The capacity of the individual to make a decision must be assessed in relation to each issue and at the time at which the decision needs to be made. For example, it cannot be assumed that a person with a learning disability lacks the capacity to make a decision on his/her current or future medical treatment, or any other aspect of his/her life, simply because at some point in the past, she or he was assessed as lacking the mental capacity to make a decision about where she or he wished to live. Nor can an individual be deemed to be incapable of making a decision simply because she or he is elderly or has been diagnosed with a condition such as a learning disability.

SECTION 3: INABILITY TO MAKE DECISIONS

Section 3 of the act sets out the criteria by which a person may be deemed to lack the mental capacity to make a decision. An individual is said to be unable to make a decision for him/herself if s/he is unable:

(a) to understand the information relevant to the decision,
(b) to retain that information,
(c) to use or weigh that information as part of the process of making the decision, or
(d) to communicate his decision (whether by talking, using sign language or any other means).

However, failure alone to understand the relevant information is not sufficient to demonstrate a lack of mental capacity. Information, especially of a legal or medical nature, can very often be presented in a language that is confusing and unintelligible to all but those in the respective profession. The act therefore requires that prior to ascertaining capacity, all information relevant to the decision should be given to the individual in a way that is appropriate to his/her circumstances, such as the use of simple language for people with learning disabilities, visual aids for people with auditory disabilities and translations for those who do not have English as their first language. It is therefore not necessary for an individual to have an in-depth technical knowledge of the issue – merely an understanding of the relevant concepts. Nor does the fact that a person is only able to retain the relevant information for a short period prevent his/her being regarded as able to make the decision. Even if an individual forgets all the information that informed his/her decision immediately after making that decision, s/he is still considered to be capable.

At this point, it is worth reiterating Key Point 3, contained in section 1 of the act: 'A person is not to be treated as unable to make a decision merely because he makes an unwise decision.' An eccentric decision that flies in the face of logic or fails to comply with the recommendation of professionals does not, in itself, constitute an absence of mental capacity. People can, and often do, make unwise decisions. People with learning disabilities have as much right to be 'wrong' as everyone else.

SECTION 4: BEST INTERESTS

Having ascertained that an individual lacks the capacity to make a decision *in relation to a specific issue or aspect of his/her life,* any decision taken on his/her behalf must be in his/her best interests. This is a term that is often used in the caring professions, with little attempt to define it. The act, however, provides a checklist of factors that decision makers must work through in deciding what is in the individual's best interest. This section of the act is one of the most comprehensive, as making decisions on somebody else's behalf is fraught with difficulty and open to abuse. In determining what is in a person's best interests, the person making the determination must not make it merely on the basis of:

(1) (a) the person's age or appearance, or
    (b) a condition of his, or an aspect of his behaviour, which might lead others to make unjustified assumptions about what might be in his best interests.
(2) The person making the determination must consider all the relevant circumstances and, in particular, take the following steps.
(3) He must consider –
    (a) whether it is likely that the person will at some time have capacity in relation to the matter in question, and
    (b) if it appears likely that he will, when that is likely to be.
(4) He must, so far as reasonably practicable, permit and encourage the person to participate, or to improve his ability to participate, as fully as possible in any act done for him and any decision affecting him.
(5) Where the determination relates to life-sustaining treatment he must not, in considering whether the treatment is in the best interests of the person concerned, be motivated by a desire to bring about his death.
(6) He must consider, so far as is reasonably ascertainable –
    (a) the person's past and present wishes and feelings (and, in particular, any relevant written statement made by him when he had capacity),
    (b) the beliefs and values that would be likely to influence his decision if he had capacity, and
    (c) the other factors that he would be likely to consider if he were able to do so.
(7) He must take into account, if it is practicable and appropriate to consult them, the views of –
    (a) anyone named by the person as someone to be consulted on the matter in question or on matters of that kind,
    (b) anyone engaged in caring for the person or interested in his welfare,
    (c) any donee of a lasting power of attorney granted by the person, and

(d) any deputy appointed for the person by the court, as to what would be in the person's best interests and, in particular, as to the matters mentioned in subsection (6).

Section 4, subsections (1)–(7) are not only intended to ensure that the 'best interests' of those assessed as lacking mental capacity are served, but that their wishes are also respected and that any decision taken on their behalf will be as close as possible to the decision that they would have made if able to do so. It should be noted, however, that there are a number of areas in which carers are still prohibited from making a decision on another's behalf, regardless of any incapacity. Even if a carer can demonstrate that it is in the best interests and compatible with the wishes of the individual, decisions about marriage, sexual relationships, adoption or voting cannot be made on behalf of another person.

LEGAL SAFEGUARDS

In order to further protect vulnerable individuals, the act also creates two new public bodies: the Court of Protection and the Public Guardian. The Court of Protection will have jurisdiction relating to the whole act and will deal with matters relating to property and serious decisions affecting health care and or welfare of individuals who lack capacity. It will also be the final arbiter in determining the capacity of an individual, where this is in doubt. The primary function of the Public Guardian is to establish and monitor a register of lasting powers of attorney. A further key provision of the act is the creation of the Independent Mental Capacity Advocate (IMCA), who will be appointed to support those individuals assessed as lacking capacity who have no one to speak for them. However, at the time of writing, there is no clear definition of their role or how the service will be organised.

CONCLUSION

At the dawn of the twentieth century, society and professionals such as Lewis Terman believed people with learning disabilities to be inherently criminal, genetically predisposed towards illegal and immoral activity. As such, the legislation of the day sought to protect society from the danger that people with learning disabilities were believed to pose. Legislation at the dawn of the twenty-first century strives to serve a similar function in that its purpose is to protect. Unlike the earlier legislation, however, the main beneficiaries this time are people with learning disabilities.

Starting with the Mental Health Act 1983 and culminating with the Disability Discrimination and Human Rights Acts, legislation in the United

Kingdom has increasingly acknowledged and embraced the rights of people with learning disabilities. Although far too early to judge the Mental Capacity Act, the barometer of existing legislation would appear to indicate that the climate for people with learning disabilities is sunnier than it has ever been.

REFERENCES

Bluglass, R. (1983) *A Guide to the Mental Health Act 1983*, Edinburgh, Churchill Livingstone.

Terman, L. M. (1916) *The Measurement of Intelligence*, Boston, Houghton Mifflin.

FURTHER READING

Brading, J. & Curtis, J. (2000) *Disability Discrimination: a Practical Guide to the New Law. 2nd Edition.* London, Kogan Page.

Hughes, A. & Coombs, P. (2001) *Easy Guide to the Human Rights Act 1998, Implications for People with Learning Disabilities.* British Institute of Learning Disabilities.

Mental Health Foundation (2005) Executive Briefing: The Mental Capacity Act. *Need2Know (1).*

The Stationery Office (1983) *Mental Health Act 1983.* Norwich: The Stationery Office.

The Stationery Office (1995) *Disability Discrimination Act 1995.* Norwich: The Stationery Office.

The Stationery Office (1998) *The Human Rights Act 1998.* Norwich: The Stationery Office.

The Stationery Office (2005) *Mental Capacity Act 2005.* Norwich: The Stationery Office.

10 Parents with Learning Disabilities

APRIL HAMMOND

KEY POINTS

- There is still a significant number of parents with learning disabilities who have had their children taken into care.
- Historically, women with mild to moderate learning disabilities were targeted and referred to as 'moral defectives', especially if they were known or thought to be sexually active.
- Discriminatory beliefs about individuals can often be based on assumptions frequently derived from historical and cultural beliefs, passed on from generation to generation.
- Many years of discrimination have made it very difficult for people with learning disabilities to prove that they have the maturity and wisdom to be good parents.

INTRODUCTION

At the turn of the twentieth century, generally, adults with learning disabilities were not considered capable of parenthood and many women with learning disabilities were incarcerated for 'immoral behaviour' (Potts & Fido 1991) in institutions or hospitals if they became pregnant out of wedlock; in most cases, the children were taken away from them.

In today's society, a more tolerant view is being promoted by services for parents with learning disabilities, with full government backing from the White Paper *Valuing People* (Department of Health 2001), although the true prevalence of these parents is unknown (Booth & Booth 1998).

However, it has been documented that there is still a significant number of parents with learning disabilities who have had their children taken into care (Booth et al. 2005), which may indicate that society may still lack confidence in trusting adults with learning disabilities to be good or even adequate parents. The reasons for this lack of confidence could be based on a variety of factors, which include unfounded, historically based prejudiced views,

Caring for People with Learning Disabilities. Edited by I. Peate and D. Fearns.
Copyright © 2006 by John Wiley & Sons, Ltd.

some of which current valuing beliefs and practices may not have totally dispelled. This may include beliefs that adults with learning disabilities may be too immature to have or develop adequate parenting skills (Thompson 2001).

Genetics and eugenics are also significant factors in a society in which genetic technology is used to determine the gender and physical status of the unborn child and deciding which children will be considered genetically acceptable and which will not, and could have a knock-on effect on society's acceptance of people with learning disabilities as parents.

Another factor is the welfare of the children whose parents have a learning disability and, in particular, any stigma or discrimination that they may suffer as a direct result of having parents with learning disabilities. This may well influence professionals involved in child protection proceedings making decisions about the suitability of adults with learning disabilities as parents and the best environment for these children to grow up in.

In this chapter, these significant factors regarding learning disabilities will be explored in more detail and case studies will be used to illustrate their impact and other relevant implications for parents with learning disabilities and their supporters.

THE HISTORICAL PERSPECTIVE

Historically, in England, there were two main themes underpinning society's attitude towards people with learning disabilities: one in which they were seen as innocent and in need of protection; and one in which they were seen as ignorant, irresponsible and promiscuous and, without proper control, could be a danger to society.

The idea that adults with learning disabilities were child-like and naive and described as 'innocents', with the inability to develop their mental capacities beyond those of children, dates back to early English history, as illustrated in this seventeenth-century legal definition:

'He has no manner of understanding or reason nor government of himself, what is for his profit or not for his profit.'

(Potts & Fido 1991)

This patronising view continued to be upheld until the mid-twentieth century and became more formally acknowledged in 1946, when a group of parents set up the National Association of Parents of Backward Children. This organisation, which would later become Mencap, promoted a child-like and vulnerable image of people with learning disabilities, who needed help, care and protection. Advocating their sons' and daughters' immature status also provided these parents with a justifiable reason for protecting their 'children' from being vilified as 'mental defectives' and being incarcerated in institutions. Unfortunately, during the early twentieth century, the other popularly held attitude about people with learning disabilities was that they needed to be controlled and segregated from society:

> '... for instigating and spreading alcoholism, prostitution and criminal activities.'
>
> (Potts & Fido 1991)

This belief was upheld more by propaganda, promoted by influential activists, than by actual criminal evidence but it still led to many individuals' being unfairly and unjustifiably incarcerated in institutions, specifically built for adults with learning disabilities.

These activists often held influential and respected positions in politics and medicine, which enabled them to promote their views, with very little opposition, debate or calls for evidence to justify such beliefs. One belief was based on the then popular eugenic ideology that focused on breeding a superior human race, which later became more notoriously associated with the atrocities carried out by the Nazis in the Second World War (Lyn 2001). Such beliefs encouraged the segregation of men and women in institutions and can be brought to life in the prejudiced words of the activist Mary Dendy (early twentieth century): '... so as to prevent, transmitting their mental and social ineptitude to their offspring ... the evil can be cured by preventing it' (cited in Wright & Digby 1996).

Women with mild to moderate learning disabilities in particular were targeted and referred to as 'moral defectives', especially if they were known or thought to be sexually active. Many of these women were placed in institutions for the duration of their child-bearing years and, in some cases, the children of these women were also incarcerated (Brigham et al. 2000). This was compounded by the belief that these children might inherit the 'learning disability' from their mothers and, in many cases, evidence was sought to substantiate this belief via the family history (Wright & Digby 1996).

History, therefore, has given adults with learning disabilities a discriminatory and questionable status in society: either they were perceived as childlike and in need of protection, or they were deemed as 'evil' and society needed to be protected from them. Neither of these characteristics could be considered conducive to parenthood. Erroneously, discrimination against adults with learning disabilities via such prejudiced views is still being sustained in society today (Thompson 2001). Even though the institutions have nearly all been closed and tremendous efforts have been made to promote the rights and equality of adults with learning disabilities, especially in the last decade, there is still sustainable evidence of discrimination towards adults with learning disabilities. This is shown in studies such as 'Health for All?' (Band 1998) – a Mencap report that revealed that people with learning disabilities were more prone to discrimination from the healthcare services than were the general population – and by reviewing child protection cases of children whose parents had learning disabilities (Booth et al. 2005).

DISCRIMINATION AND DIVERSITY

Discriminatory beliefs about individuals can often be based on assumptions frequently derived from historical and cultural beliefs, passed on from generation to generation. Through this process, many discriminatory beliefs become enmeshed in society's infrastructure and can become acceptable and commendable or even lead to radical actions, like the termination of a foetus with a disability (legally accepted in the Abortion Act 1967).

Discriminatory assumptions against people with learning disabilities need to be better understood before being condemned or disregarded, especially if society is to be expected to be less discriminatory in its behaviour towards these individuals (Thompson 2001). In particular, for adults with learning disabilities who become or wish to become parents, the perception that they can be seen as 'child-like' needs to be better understood. Initially, this perception was probably derived from an intention to be protective towards individuals who, due to their reduced cognitive abilities or limited speech, were seen as vulnerable and unable to fend for themselves. Further protection could be given if they were dressed in children's clothes and labelled as asexual and incapable of sexual feelings. Even the activists who promoted institutional care considered that they were protecting vulnerable people from society, as much as protecting society from them. The belief that people with learning disabilities need protection is still being upheld in some contemporary communities, with the majority of people with learning disabilities still living in supervised environments. Further justification can be given for this via reports of abusive and exploitive behaviours and attitudes towards individuals who live more independently in the community, such as the significant numbers of rape and sexual abuse cases reported against women with learning disabilities (Crossmaker 1991; McCarthy 1999; Parkes 2003).

PARENTING

Traditionally, the role of a parent is seen predominately as an adult one, not suited to children. So, for people with learning disabilities, the discriminatory connotations associated with their being child-like can be further complicated by beliefs that it is not appropriate for children to take on a parenting role. Reder et al. (2000) saw parenthood as 'Not an activity which sits comfortably within the paradigm of childhood as constitutes the child's appropriate role and place in the adult world'. This indicates that if an adult with a learning disability is considered to be child-like in behaviour, then assumptions about the ability of this adult to be a parent could be made based on assumptions of a child's ability to be a parent. This assumption also implies that before an adult with a learning disability can be considered as suitable to be a parent, s/he must first be seen as an adult. This then leads to questioning what adult qualities and behaviours contribute towards an acceptable paradigm of parenting. The *Oxford Thesaurus* (1994) describes being an adult as being seen as being mature, sensible, grown up, responsible, wise, prepared and ready. These admirable qualities have not, historically, been attributed to people with learning disabilities. The role of a parent has also been described as 'One of the most valued social roles in Western Society' (Woodhouse et al. 2001), whereas having a learning disability is probably still considered one of the least socially valued attributes to have in today's society. Years of discrimination and prevention, either with or without good intentions, have made it very difficult for people with learning disabilities to prove that they have the maturity and wisdom to be good parents. When opportunities for people with learning disabilities to be parents did arise, all too often, a decision on their behalf was made to prevent this happening.

The following case study illustrates how such a decision was made for a young woman with learning disabilities.

Case study

A young woman, who had a severe learning disability and could not communicate verbally, was placed in an institution in the late 1940s as a child when her parents were advised it would be best for her, as it was assumed she would never behave like an adult and would always need to be looked after. She grew up in a single-sex ward and her parents visited her until they died. She gradually developed more independent skills, but did not learn to talk. As a young woman, she used to walk to and from her ward to the day unit, independently. She appeared happy in her own way but it was noted that she did not have any particular friends in the institution. It was a total shock to the staff when she was found to be approximately five months' pregnant and unable to explain how it happened. A few months later, she was taken to the local hospital to give birth and then brought back to the institution, whilst the baby remained in the hospital, awaiting adoption. The staff were very supportive towards her in the hospital but reported that it was a terrible experience for her, as she was still just like a 'child' herself. Afterwards, she was given a daily oral contraceptive pill and continued to walk alone to and from the day unit. The father of the child was never identified. Nothing more was reported about the baby and it is unknown what she was told about the baby.

Ten years later, she moved to a residential home and began a new life in the community. Many years later, an Advocate tried, unsuccessfully, to locate further information about the baby and the father.

Consider the following:

- How would a young woman of the same age, with a learning disability, who became pregnant, be viewed by today's society?
- How would a young woman of the same age, but without a learning disability, who became pregnant, be viewed by today's society?
- What, historically, might have affected the actions of the care staff?

EUGENICS AND ETHICAL ISSUES

History, unfortunately, for adults with learning disabilities is not the only barrier standing between them and their credible status as parents or potential parents. The science of genetics has impacted on society's tolerance towards people with learning disabilities by providing parents-to-be with a means to determine whether their unborn children with disabilities live or not. Parents-to-be can choose not to give birth to seriously disabled babies, as clarified in the Abortion Act 1967, in which it states that it:

'Will not be unlawful ... if there is substantial risk that if the child were born it would suffer from such physical or mental abnormalities as to be seriously handicapped.'

There are up to 100 conditions detectable in the womb (Hernstein & Murray 1994) and over 90 per cent of those who know that their foetus has Down's syndrome terminate the pregnancy (Ward 2001). Such figures bring to mind the consideration of ethical issues such as: Will parents who choose to have the disabled child feel discriminated against? And will there be further implications for adults with learning disabilities who are, or who wish to become, parents? Genetic screening has also evoked eugenic values, as demonstrated in China, where, in 1994, a eugenic screening programme was introduced to reduce the number of 'inferior births' (Ward 2001). There are concerning issues, too, regarding how human characteristics are defined and valued in society and who makes those decisions on which characteristics are valued and which are not. Also, eugenic beliefs are still being sanctioned in current literature, as cited by Lyn (2001), who maintains that 'The belief in the eugenic objectives of eliminating genetic diseases, increasing intelligence and reducing personality disorders remain desirable'.

However, genetic counselling and technology, although often used as a means to assist in determining the characteristics of the unborn child, cannot be held accountable for how the characteristics are valued and whether or not a child will be born. In fact, genetic counselling can also be perceived in more positive ways, such as enabling parents to seek out information and support prior to the birth and by providing evidence that not all learning disability characteristics are genetically based.

The following case study considers the genetic issues that might affect a married couple who have learning disabilities.

Case study

A couple, who both have mild learning disabilities, lived in a residential home, fell in love and married. They were then supported to live in their own flat in the community. After five years of marriage, they decided they wanted children and each had expressed this wish independently to their support worker.

The support worker, however, is concerned, as the wife has Down's syndrome and she wonders whether or not the child might have Down's syndrome and whether the couple will be able to cope with this.

- What advice, if any, should the support worker give this couple?
- How might the couple feel if they are advised to seek genetic counselling?
- Is the support worker valuing their wishes?

How people with learning disabilities are valued in society is still greatly debated by people with learning disabilities, their families and service providers. Since the closure of the institutions and the implementation of the Care in the Community Act 1989 and the White Paper *Valuing People* (Department of Health 2001), there has been a considerable and positive change in the welfare of people with learning disabilities in all areas of their lives. However, it has also been acknowledged that people with learning disabilities are still being under-valued and discriminated against (O'Hara & Martin 2003) and one area in which this appears prevalent is the way in which parents with learning disabilities are perceived, particularly by the services that support them (Booth et al. 2005; Woodhouse et al. 2001).

CARING FOR CHILDREN

The discussion above may be the result of the implementation of the Children Act 1989, in which a greater emphasis has been placed on the protection of children who are considered vulnerable and are consequently being placed on the 'At Risk Register'. This legally requires that:

'The register should list all the children resident in the area who are considered to be at continuing risk of significant harm and for whom there is a child protection plan.'

(Children Act 1989)

The local authorities have the statutory duty to investigate all children who live in, or are found in, their area who are considered to be suffering or likely to suffer significant harm (Children Act 1989). The local authorities also have the power to provide services for children at risk and their families. However, Parton (1997), in reviewing the effectiveness of the children's services, found there to be a narrow focus on abuse and child protection, with more cases being put on the register without enough family support systems being implemented. So parents whose children were on the register might feel stigmatised but not supported by the local authorities.

Significantly, parents who have learning disabilities are more likely to have their children placed on the register than any other parent group and a service audit in the United Kingdom stated that 93 per cent of children born to parents with learning disabilities had interventions via child protection (Woodhouse et al. 2001). Another survey revealed that 40 per cent of children born to English mothers with learning disabilities were put into care, long-term fostering or were adopted following child protection proceedings (O'Hara & Martin 2003).

The most common reason for children to be placed under child protection is neglect (Butler & Roberts 2004).

Neglect, as stated by the Children Act 1989, is said to be:

'. . . the persistent failure to meet a child's basic physical and psychological needs, likely to result in the serious impairment of the child's health or development. Parent/carer fails to provide adequate food, shelter and clothing, failing to protect from physical harm or danger, failing to ensure access to appropriate medical and treatment. It may also include neglect of a child's basic emotional needs.'

(Children Act 1989)

Some of these 'negligent' behaviours, especially the emotional ones, may be difficult or too vague to classify. For many adults with learning disabilities, these ambiguous terms can be used to make judgements by professionals on their parenting abilities, even before their children are born. Booth et al. (2005) found, on surveying Child Protection Reports, that a significantly high number of newborn babies whose mothers had learning disabilities were being presented at Court Protection hearings. This prediction has been further borne out in studies that reveal that parents with learning disabilities have been discriminated against and viewed as neglectful through simple misunderstandings, such as being seen to be deliberately avoiding child care appointments when actually they were unaware of the appointments because they could not read the invitations (O'Hara & Martin 2003).

However, other studies have revealed significant figures of child abuse by parents with learning disabilities (Feldman 1986; Whitman & Accardo 1990). Many parents with learning disabilities have also been found to be living in poverty and social isolation, thus reducing their opportunities to learn parenting skills through appropriate social contacts such as attending school functions and mixing with other parents (Woodhouse et al. 2001).

The children of parents with learning disabilities can also become victims, even if their parents are providing good care. As the children grow up and become aware of their parents' disabilities, they may develop protective roles towards their parents and, in some cases, even become their parents' carer (Booth & Booth 1998). Many of these children have reported difficulties in their early lives and have suffered bullying from their peers (Crabtree & Warner 1999). Despite this, there is some anecdotal evidence which reports many children (both as children and adults) of parents with learning disabilities describing deep feelings of closeness and love towards their parents (Bibby & Becker 2000; Booth & Booth 1998). This view is further reinforced in a study carried out by Perkins et al. (2002) on the emotional well-being of children whose parents have learning disabilities which revealed that the children were more able to cope with the stigma of having a parent with a learning disability if the relationship between parent and child was warm and loving.

PROVISION OF SUPPORT

A steadily increasing number of parents with learning disabilities are being referred to social and health services for support and advice in parenting skills, although there are no reliable estimates of the number of parents with learning disabilities residing in Britain (Booth & Booth 1998). Added to this, more people with learning disabilities are experiencing greater opportunities to choose how they wish to live, since it has been officially acknowledged that they have the same rights as others through the Human Rights Act 1998, The Disability Discrimination Act 1995 and the White Paper *Valuing People* (Department of Health 2001). However, the Law Commission (1995) reported that 'Community living has exposed many vulnerable people to new or at least different dangers, when they are put at risk by being allowed to live their lives as they choose'.

It is still not known how effectively the principles and ethos underpinning *Valuing People* (Department of Health 2001) will work in a practical way in supporting people with learning disabilities to be valued citizens living in the community. What is known is that some adults with learning disabilities will choose not to be identified with the label 'learning disabilities' or 'learning difficulties' and attempt to live under 'A cloak of competence', as described by Edgerton (1997). Edgerton surveyed a group of people with learning disabilities discharged from an institution in America and found that the majority of women wanted to marry 'normal' men and free themselves from any public discrimination associated with their past. Nunkoosing and John (1997) revealed similar views when they carried out a survey about relationships and feelings with a group of people with learning disabilities in England.

It may be understandable, considering the level of discrimination that people with learning disabilities have endured over the years, that some may choose not to look for support, for fear of discrimination and loss of control in their lives; furthermore, some parents with learning disabilities may equally fear that they will be discriminated against and their children will be removed and may be wary of asking for help, even if they would benefit from it.

The following case study illustrates how a mother tried to manage when the school reported that her daughter was not eating school dinners.

Case study

The family consisted of Mum, with moderate learning disabilities, Dad with borderline learning disabilities and a 7-year-old daughter who did not have a learning disability. They all lived in a neat and well kept two-bedroomed house.

The family managed without outside support and did not normally mix with their neighbours, but, recently, Mum had been befriended by a lady who had just moved into the neighbourhood. One day, Mum received a note from her daughter's school, which normally she would ask her husband to read but as he was out, she asked her new friend and neighbour to read. The note raised concerns that her daughter was not eating her school dinners and wished her parents to be aware of the situation. After the note was read to her, Mum confessed to her friend that she was still spoon-feeding her daughter at home and thought that the daughter might expect the teachers to do the same at school. She was not too concerned, as her daughter was not under-weight and she explained to the neighbour that her daughter would help herself to biscuits when she thought her mum and dad were not looking. Her neighbour reassured her that there was nothing to worry about and that it was likely the daughter would soon start eating independently, as she seemed a bright and happy child.

The neighbour then went straight home and reported the parents to the local authority, stating that she thought the mother was unfit to be a mother, due to her learning disabilities.

Consequently, the whole family were referred, via the local authority, to the Learning Disability Team. Whilst they were carrying out an assessment, they found out that the parents had never asked for or received any formal support in helping to raise their daughter, and they were very reluctant to engage with the team for fear that their daughter might be taken away.

The daughter remained with her parents and eventually they accepted the support of a carer provided by the team.

- What might have influenced the parents to fear that their daughter would be taken away?
- Was the local authority obliged to respond to the neighbour's concerns?
- Was the neighbour acting in the best interests of the daughter or discriminating against the mother?

The Government has stated that 'The rights of people with learning disabilities to have a family is at the heart of the strategy "Valuing People"' (Department of Health 2001), yet it was noted by O'Hara and Martin (2003) that there are few integrated and coordinated services to meet their needs.

However, there is now some hope being offered to parents with learning disabilities through the Sure Start schemes that are being set up as part of the Government's 10-year strategy for child care, which has intentions of closing:

'The gap in outcomes between the disadvantaged and their peers, as well as promoting diversity and addressing social exclusion through the provision of support.'

(DfES & DWP 2004)

This report has further outlined how parents will be included in ensuring that the services meet their needs as well as the needs of their children. So it is to be hoped that this will improve the services for parents who have learning disabilities. When services have been designed and implemented specifically for parents with learning disabilities, they have proved to be successful in promoting and improving parenting skills and reducing the number of children taken into care. Such services have provided support, information and a suitable environment in which to develop skills, given parents the right to show responsibility and demonstrate their own abilities, and provided further workshops for parents, parents-to-be and professionals (Brickley 2003; Woodhouse et al. 2001).

Parents with learning disabilities have also expressed being able to cope better if they are supported in a non-judgemental way and given specific help with tasks that they may feel unable to do themselves, such as helping their children with their school work (Atkinson et al. 2000), and by being supported in their own homes (Llewellyn et al. 2002). Parents with learning disabilities have also felt more able to voice their fears and feelings if they believe that they will be listened to and not judged as being unsuited to being parents:

'The best thing about being a parent is that you have a lot of fun out of them . . . you can play with them . . . tickle them and have a good conversation with them.'

(The views of a mother with learning disabilities, who was interviewed, Atkinson et al. 2000)

CONCLUSION

There is hope for the future for parents with learning disabilities and adults with learning disabilities who wish to become parents, if the current specific support services continue to deliver the quality of support and commitment that they are already providing and if the government continues with its commitment to supporting and protecting parents, as well as children, from discrimination.

Parents with learning disabilities will also need the commitments outlined in *Valuing People* (Department of Health 2001) to continue to impact positively on the welfare and services provided for people with learning disabilities. Finally, it is to be hoped that parents with learning disabilities will be able to shake off their past devaluing image and become truly valued as members of society and accepted as good parents if they are good parents.

REFERENCES

Atkinson, D., Mcarthy, M., Walmsey, J., Cooper, M., Rolfe, S., Aspis, S., et al. (2000) *Good Times, Bad Times; Women with Learning Difficulties Telling their Stories*, Kidderminster, Bild Publications.

Band, R. (1998) *The NHS: Health for All?*, a Mencap report, Mencap.

Bibby, A. & Becker, S. (eds) (2000) *Young Carers in their Own Words*, London, Calouste Gulbenkian Foundation.

Booth, T. & Booth, W. (1998) *Growing up with Parents Who Have Learning Difficulties*, London, Routledge.

Booth, T., Booth, W. & McConnell, D. (2005) 'The Prevalence and Outcomes of Care Proceedings Involving Parents with Learning Difficulties in the Family Courts', *Journal of Applied Research in Intellectual Disabilities*, **18**(1): 7–17.

Brickley, S. (2003) 'Working with Parents Who Have a Learning Disability and their Children', in M. Jukes & M. Bollard (eds), *Contemporary Learning Disability Practice*, Salisbury, MA Healthcare Limited.

Brigham, L., Atkinson, D., Jackson, M., Rolph, S. & Walmsey, J. (2000) *Crossing Boundaries: Change and Continuity in the History of Learning Disability*, Kidderminster, BILD Publications.

Butler, I. & Roberts, G. (2004) *Social Work with Children and Families: Getting into Practice*, 2nd edn, London/New York, Jessica Kingsley Publishers.

Crabtree, H. & Warner, L. (1999) *Too Much to Take On: A Report on Young Carers and Bullying*, The Princess Royal Trust for Carers.

Crossmaker, M. (1991) 'Behind Closed Doors: Institutional Sexual Abuse', *Sexuality and Disability*, **9**(3): 210–19.

Department of Health (2001) *Valuing People: A New Strategy for Learning Disability for the 21st Century*, London, HMSO.

DfES & DWP (2004) *Choice for Parents, the Best Start for Children*, London, HMSO.

Edgerton, R. (1997) *A Cloak of Competence*, Berkley/Los Angeles/London, University of California Press.

Feldman, M. A. (1986) 'Research of Parenting of Mentally Retarded Persons', *Psychiatric Clinical North America*, **9**: 777, also in M. Jukes & M. Bollard (2003) *Contemporary Learning Disability Practice*, Salisbury, MA Healthcare Limited, Chapter 5, pp. 51–61.

Hernstein, R. J. & Murray, C. (1994) *The Bell Curve: Intelligence and Class Structure in American Life*, New York, Free Press.

Law Commission (1995) *Mental Incapacity Law*, Com. No. 231, HMSO.

Llewellyn, G., McConnell, D., Russo, D., Mayes, R. & Honey, A. (2002) 'Home-Based Programmes for Parents with Intellectual Disabilities: Lessons from Practice', *Journal of Applied Research in Intellectual Disabilities*, **15**(4): 341–53.

Lyn, R. (2001) *Eugenics: A Reassessment*, Westport, CT, Praeger/Greenwood.

McCarthy, M. (1999) *Sexuality and Women with Learning Disabilities*, Tyne and Wear, Athenaeum Press.

Nunkoosing, K. & John, M. (1997) 'Friendship, Relationships and the Management of Rejection and Loneliness by People with Learning Disabilities', *Journal of Learning Disabilities for Nursing Health and Social Care*, **1**(1): 10–18.

O'Hara, J. & Martin, H. (2003) 'Parents with Learning Disabilities: A Study of Gender and Cultural Perspectives in East London', *British Journal of Learning Disabilities*, **31**(1): 18–24.

Oxford Thesaurus (1994) Oxford University Press.

Parkes, N. (2003) 'Abuse and Vulnerability', in M. Jukes & M. Bollard (eds), *Contemporary Learning Disability Practice*, Salisbury, Quay Books, pp. 151–64.

Parton, N. (1997) *Child Protection and Family Support: Tensions, Contradictions and Possibilities*, London, Routledge.

Perkins, T. S., Holburn, S., Deaux, K., Flory, M. J. & Vietze, P. M. (2002) 'Children of Mothers with Intellectual Disability: Stigma, Mother–Child Relationship and Self-Esteem', *Journal of Applied Research in Intellectual Disabilities*, **15**(4): 297–313.

Potts, M. & Fido, R. (1991) *A Fit Person to be Removed*, Plymouth Northgate House Publishers Ltd.

Reder, P., McClure, M. & Jolley, A. (eds) (2000) *Family Matters: Interfaces between Child and Adult Mental Health*, London, Routledge, p. 5.

Thompson, N. (2001) *Anti-Discriminatory Practice*, 3rd edn, Basingstoke, Palgrave.

Ward, L. (2001) *Considered Choices? The New Genetics, Prenatal Testing and People with Learning Disabilities*, Kidderminster, BILD Publications.

Whitman, B. & Accardo, P. J. (1990) *When a Parent is Mentally Retarded*, Baltimore, Brookes.

Woodhouse, A. E., Green, G. & Davies, S. (2001) 'Parents with Learning Disabilities: Service Audit and Development', *British Journal of Learning Disabilities*, **29**: 128–32.

Wright, D. & Digby, A. (1996) *From Idiocy to Mental Deficiency: Historical Perspectives of People with Learning Disabilities*, London, Routledge.

Index

Caring for People with Learning Disabilities. Edited by I. Peate and D. Fearns.
Copyright © 2006 by John Wiley & Sons, Ltd.